MW00876103

Walk In Balance

**A personal energy guide for busy people everywhere
to be their Best in the 21st Century**

*Resolving the Energy depletion issue so many face today -
Focusing, Filling up your feel good Energy-Wellness tank,
Living your life fully, making a Difference
in the most efficient Balanced way possible ...*

by
William Jason O'Mara

with
Sybrian Castleman

January 2016

www.walkinbalance.org

Library of Congress Data

O'Mara, William Jason, 1962 -
Walk In Balance

By WJ O'Mara Phd

ISBN-13:978-1516988082
ISBN-10: 1516988086
1. Spiritual Life. 2. Self Help

Manuscript editor
April Rowe: april.rwe@gmail.com
Liesbeth Leysen: liesbeth.leysen.mol@gmail.com

Printed in the United States by

William Jason O'Mara, 2007, 2016

Address all inquiries to:

Bill@walkinbalance.org
Sybrian@walkinbalance.org

www.WalkinBalance.org

Disclaimer:
This book, should not be considered, in any way,
to replace sound professional medical or
psychological consultation and/or treatment.

On Facebook at: www.facebook.com/WalknBalance

Acknowledgments

Bill
My deepest gratitude and heartfelt thank you to Patrick Edward Quirk (Speaking Wind); and to all my teachers, friends and family for their support, lessons, and love as I go through my own journey in life. A special Thank you goes to all of the readers in the early stages who offered important feedback. Thank you so much Liesbeth Leysen for you. Thank you Sybrian and Mac for your wonderful WIB sharing.

Thank you to Wayne Dyer, Marianne Williamson, James Redfield, Stuart Wilde, and others whose books have kept me inspired for many years with progressive teachings.

In addition, thank you to the countless friends and strangers who offered me kind words, hope, and lessons during my travels. My appreciation also goes to Starwood Hotels, CFLG, Kripalu Center, Ojai Foundation, and Esalen for creating wonderful organizations that truly serve humanity.

Sybrian
I am very thankful to Rich Rowe (of the *American Advancement Institute*). There are many experiences and opportunities I sought due to the inspiration and encouragement he provided.

Immense gratitude goes to my mentor of many years, Major L. Roy Lynch (of *USAF Auxiliary/Civil Air Patrol*). He will be forever missed in my life and the lives of many others who he influenced through his dedication, humor, and teachings in aviation, leadership, nature, and Native American wisdom.

I am deeply grateful for each and every one of you who have been a part of my life. Thank you for sharing my journey.

This book is about exploring your life, there is no One way.
Pull from a variety of ways, and create what works for you in your
personal "Walk in Balance" plan.

Walk In Balance SHIFT Work -

Want to integrate the lessons of this Book more deeply in your day to day life, one on one personally with one of the authors?

It's now available.

Ask us about Shift Coaching to help you Walk In Balance.

www.WalkinBalance.org

bill@walkinbalance.org
sybrian@walkinbalance.org

Table of Contents

Wild Geese

You do not have to be good.
You do not have to walk on your knees
For a hundred miles through the desert, repenting.
You only have to let the soft animal of your body
love what it loves.

Tell me about your despair, yours, and I will tell you mine.
Meanwhile the world goes on.
Meanwhile the sun and the clear pebbles of the rain
are moving across the landscapes,
over the prairies and the deep trees,
the mountains and the rivers.

Meanwhile the wild geese, high in the clean blue air,
are heading home again.
Whoever you are, no matter how lonely,
the world offers itself to your imagination,
calls to you like the wild geese, harsh and exciting --
over and over announcing your place
in the family of things.

- *Mary Oliver*

I Will Not Die an Unlived Life

I will not die an unlived life.
I will not live in fear
of falling or catching fire.
I choose to inhabit my days,
to allow my living to open me,
to make me less afraid,
more accessible,
to loosen my heart
until it becomes a wing,
a torch, a promise.
I choose to risk my significance.
to live so that which came to me as blossom,
goes on as fruit.

- *Dawna Markova*

Opening Meditation

Say a gentle prayer
Enter sacred space

Find your heart
Be

Fill your tank with the sunlight
Breathing in - I calm my mind and body
Breathing out - I release and I trust

The Peace of God is my only Goal
All is well in my world

Love all around us
Deep bow,
Thank you.

Introduction

This is not a book on time management or the like per se. It is a deep look at all facets of our lives. This book can help you identify a very personal Life plan (map) and living practices that can help you live the way you want to live and be your best.

It starts with asking, "Who am I and what do I want?" It then deepens to add daily self-nourishment 'energy' practices to help you feel happy and alive. These are choices, not prescriptions. As such they become 'self-chosen' disciplines we can practice each day with joy, like an Olympian in training, to help us live the successful journey.

This life plan is not a plan in the traditional sense. It's not an intellectual thing, or a dogma, or a list of beliefs. It is not about changing everything or quitting your job, or what we 'must' do. It's simply whatever we want from soul, to help you live authentically, freely, fully alive. This is experiential augmentation: waking up to new possibilities, choosing to feel good, walking a new walk, playing, learning what we love, practicing, and living what our soul calls for and for no other reason than we want to live a joyful life.

So if a particular exercise in life doesn't fill you (even though someone else loves it, or recommends it), don't do it. (Jogging, for example.) Find another exercise that is joyful for you. Fear not, many of us have major responsibilities right now. Take care of them, just give yourself time to renew, refresh, explore, and see where it goes. Trust. Do what fills you, and see.

My conviction is that with a little time, you can create this balance, and live the life you have imagined a bit more each year of life. Hence, see this book as your life handbook; walk with it, journal with it; make the choices your soul is calling you to make. As you do, the adventure of all adventures begins. We dream a new dream. It comes true and life is better than we could have believed.

So, let's listen to you and create the life you want. No one can do it for you. The universe awaits your decision. And as you do.... living the way you want to live, being the best human spirit you can, you become an example to support others in their evolution. We can thus help others by helping ourselves.

~Bill

Sybrian and Mac having Lunch...

Mac: Sybrian you look so great... What have you been doing lately to look so great?

Sybrian: I told you Mac, you just never listen!

Mac: You mean that Walk in Balance with O'Mara again? I'm so tired of that malarkey!

Sybrian: Its only malarkey if you really go for it and it doesn't work for you, Mac!

Mac: Yeah, Yeah, Yeah. I'm tired of Gurus.

Sybrian: It's not about any Guru. It's about YOU Mac.

Mac: What do you mean?

Sybrian: You constantly complain, and feel lousy, and never have any energy... right?

Mac: Yeah, I guess I so....

Sybrian: So, would you like to feel better? It's that simple.

Mac: Of course! But it's not "that simple".
I have tried everything. I exercise, I eat right, but I'm dragging all the time.

Sybrian: Exercise and good food is a start. But bottom line, Trying things doesn't work.
Mac: What do you mean?

Sybrian: Do you ever try to feel better?

Mac: Yeah.

Sybrian: What happens?

Mac: Nothing.
Sybrian: Exactly!!

Mac: So, what am I supposed to do?

Sybrian: You've got to go for it, Mac!
When are you going to do it? I mean, really DO it?

Mac: I don't know.

Sybrian: Mac, you're not getting any younger. The time to do it....is
NOW. You want to feel great, look great, get stuff done, enjoy
yourself....right?

Mac: Right.

Sybrian: You want a balanced life...right?

Mac: I do, but....

Sybrian: But what? What's holding you back?

Mac: I'm scared to go for it again. No matter what I do in any part
of my life, I just seem to fail. Every time.

Sybrian: What else?

Mac: I'm just tired of it all. I've tried so much, so many times, and
nothing ever works for me.

Sybrian: I hear you. I used to feel exactly the same way. Nothing
was working for me either.

Mac: So....

Sybrian: So....How about this? Just let all the past go...drop it all behind you. You have so much talent and so much to give, but you can't get anywhere or do much when you feel so depleted and defeated.

Mac: I don't know if I can do it.

Sybrian: I'll help you. How about giving it a chance?

Mac: I can't be any worse off than I am right now. And you'll help?

Sybrian: Sure, we all need some support from our friends. Are you ready to give it a go?

Mac: You know, seeing you looking and feeling so great....Yep. You're right. I'm ready. So, where do we start?

Sybrian: It's simple. Get the book, Walk In Balance....and do it. We'll go through it together.

Mac: Okay. It might take a few days.

Sybrian: Oh, no. We're not going with that "excuse" route. Here, borrow mine and give it back when you get yours. Okay?

Mac: "Excuse" route?

Sybrian: Yep. The one where you keep meaning to get the book, but something always comes up, so it doesn't happen. You said you were ready to start, so let's start! Right now, no delays. Okay?

Mac: Okay.

Sybrian: Great! Now, the first thing we're going to need is a map.

Mac: A map?

Sybrian: Yes. A map! In life, we need a map. Not THE Map; Just a map to help guide us to where we want to be. Walk In Balance is exactly that. From it, we create our own life map and use it. It's simple. It works for me. Now, let's find out how we can make it work for you.

Mac: Okay.

Sybrian: So…Mac….Do you want to feel great, get back in balance AND get stuff done in less time with more fun? Are you ready?

Mac: YES!

The Journey

One day you finally knew what you had to do, and began,
though the voices around you kept shouting their bad advice -
though the whole house began to tremble and you felt the old
tug at your ankles. "Mend my life!" each voice cried.

But you didn't stop. You knew what you had to do,
though the wind pried with its stiff fingers at the very
foundations, though their melancholy was terrible.
It was already late enough, and a wild night,
and the road full of fallen branches and stones.

But little by little, as you left their voices behind, the stars began
to burn through the sheets of clouds, and there was a new voice
which you slowly recognized as your own,
that kept you company as you strode deeper and deeper
into the world, determined to do the only thing you could do --
determined to save the only life you could save.

- Mary Oliver

Chapter 1: The Journey

Are you on the Journey? Are you learning? What have you learned about what you need to be, to be YOUR Best? Do you take care of yourself or are you running 1000 miles per hour to who knows where/in a world of 10,000 distractions?

Taking care of ourselves is prerequisite to taking care of others, worldly success, etc. Today more than ever people are not feeling right. If we're honest, stress, disease, low energy, unhappiness, and depression touches us all in some way - and impacts our work, our relationships, and our joy.

If you have come to this book, you are wanting to know how to overcome some of these issues in order to balance your life and be maximally effective and happy.

The key with any such pursuit is... what is your priority, what do you want, and what will REALLY support you in getting there?

For me (Bill), I have noticed a big change in mè of late. As I have been exploring my mission for the journey ahead, and I have been noticing a profound shift. Meaning, I see a movement from external to internal focus; to embracing, enjoying, and seizing each beautiful moment instead of obtaining a long list of desires, which experience has taught me never really changed my state of happiness. The priorities I once longed for: success, notoriety, fame, etc. are fading. Something deeper inside is emerging, with a tear of gratitude, just enjoy this gift of life. It is a miracle you know..?

Of course, I/we all may have goals for income, travel, contribution and such. It's just something has shifted to the inside, to soul, to how I feel first, and then the rest flows with grace and inspired action. Do you follow? I found this to be vital to my life to just let go, to live, and trust the rest; give where my soul guided me to.

I would suggest the journey of our life begins, right now, one step at a time. Wherever you are, in the mud, the pain, the challenge, do your best to embrace it... and begin to imagine...to create what you want your life to be. Then we do what we know (part grace, part action); doing our very best to create our vision, to be happy.

I am a person on this same journey just like you. I sweat, cry, and have good days and bad. It's quite a ride here on earth especially at this time of quickening. I have learned from life and many teachers, I have gifts to share, about the path, about walking in balance. So I am sharing. My prayer in this book is you will learn more about you, what you want, and how to be your best you, how to come fully alive.

My writings often come from the challenges I am going through. Over the past few years leading up to this book, I found myself grappling with a fundamental human/existential paradox, one that has kept me up many a night searching. This pursuit has stretched me to the extent of my human understanding. I didn't have an answer. My upbringing didn't provide one. So I prayed intently, meditated, and explored it.

My question was, 'How do I best live on this planet, for the short time I have in a way that serves others and is life enhancing for me?' "How am I to use my precious time here to be my best?" At the root my question emerged as: "Am I to invest in being/surrender/a simpler downsized life or doing/acting/achieving in the world?" There are so many teachings, so many ways.

Some are driven to make millions of dollars as their goal; others work as social workers to help the world in some way. Others are inspired to live "off the grid" in simple/farm centric ways. My upbringing (raised in suburban NY USA 1970s) gave me long lists of what I should be doing: go for it, achieve, and get the gold. But very few of the people, I saw, who have achieved 'it' seem fulfilled, including myself. So...then what? What is true? Have you ever experienced this confusion?

Often I had answered this question of where do I put my time, with: "Is there something I am to do for the world, like 'save the world'?" So I have pursued many projects enthusiastically, working and sweating to achieve something to assist humanity. Only to find myself externalizing, working feverishly to make changes "out there" and quickly find myself way out of balance, feeling exhausted, tired, and unfulfilled. But why? Isn't service supposed to fill me up? These 'projects' were such important missions, I thought.

We could certainly argue here in the west, that we are achievement obsessed. With this obsession, the USA has some of the highest, if not the highest rates in the world for: depression, ADD, drug addiction, alcoholism, malnutrition, obesity, child abuse, and murder. How can this be? Not a pretty picture. It's very much out of balance. I can tell you I have coached many an executive who has cried in my office disgusted with how out of balance their lives have become. It's humbling.

My teacher, Native American speaker-healer Patrick Edward Quirk (*Speaking Wind*), would ask those of us at his talks to "wake up from our obsession with trying to change the world". He would say, "Stop saving the whales, and the earth, and the ozone layers and instead wake up the humans who are the ones hurting everything! Start with yourself." True.

Over the years, I started to listen. I felt so much out of balance with how I was living. I started slowly to awaken from the trance of what I was taught. I noticed all the drain and un-fulfillment of trying to save everything/one and/or achieve all the time, keep up with the Jones'. So I wondered, "Why do I want to save the world/help others? What am I trying to achieve?"

What was the reason, truly? Certainly, we can all contribute in many ways. There is so much of a need. Yet, as a dear friend once told me, Life cannot just be about out there, work or service to others. Life is also about 'in here' - our personal journey with Self, doing whatever it is that makes us truly centered, happy, balanced and alive inside (regardless if it is making anyone else happy). We don't seem to get enough of this message. We don't let ourselves be, explore, walk, laugh, play the guitar, and doing things we just love without a goal. Our self-worth is so much tied to what we are doing or achieving, or what we are giving to others. Can't we just find what we enjoy expressing-experiencing in our heart, do that, and be good with it?

Since we are here a short time, why not identify and do exactly what it is that feeds you, what you truly love, what IS priority (before the years fly by)? Even if you may not know, keep asking. One step at a time, let the new, the true arise in you. Give yourself permission to discover. Isn't it time?

Maybe for many of you, you are doing exactly what you love. You're not here to revamp everything, but to make a few new distinctions, make a few tweaks, make a few more dollars to support your children or similar (for sometimes we can be out of balance in taking too much time for being, when we could be creating something magical). All good. The question is what am I really after? To feel more energized, more connected, more alive? Why not take a new path and Walk in Balance? Join us...

Let's start with putting aside our traditional list of needs and wants, of what we were taught was right and ask inside, what turns you on? What are you here to express, to learn, to grow, to experience, and be, regardless of where it will get you and regardless of all the outside demands of the world that are so easy to get caught up in. Even if it's a few minutes a day, explore it. Don't let life pass you by doing what you 'thought' was right. Remember, "your thought" of what is right, may have been programmed by society (what to think).

We don't have to do what we think we have to do. So take the steps. Try something else, have a little faith. I meet many people going through this transition, who are moving toward how they want to live. And do you know what? They're all happier and making enough money to support themselves, their kids, etc. The universe provides when we follow the urgings of our true Self. We just need to take the step. My guess is something inside you is calling you to do so, that the old must go.

I believe we all must answer these fundamental questions, or someday we may wake up and wonder, where did my life go? I am in midlife and if you are too, this is a big part of it, to question, to discover, what have you never allowed in you? I have seen many people, even in my own family, get caught in the madness of 'should', and never explore the unlived life, which leads to regret and self-loathing. So isn't it time? Time to find out, what is the reason you are here, from the inside? What is the right balance of living for you?

This is the key chord struck, I believe, in Elizabeth Gilbert's mega best seller, 'Eat Pray Love'. Where she struggled to give herself permission to stop and take time away to unravel from her list of shoulds-musts and have to's (under much criticism from others I might add)... to reflect, question, and find her true joy self (and consequently a greater success than she could have imagined). Such courage. All of us face this initiation to "will you be you?" Or be what others say you should be?

There are many stories like Ms. Gilbert's, for there is a fundamental disconnect in the USA. The so called richest place in the world is in many ways devoid of Joy. We in the States, again have some of the highest rates of addiction, depression, abuse, mental illness, and violence in the world.

Now why is this? Think about what has happened. What is being taught to young people in our culture? In our view, it is no longer sustainable to teach shame, guilt, win at all costs competition, and so forth inherent in our ways.

There is another way: A more conscious path. One for you, which you choose that best fills you; and the one that most connects to your spirit and joy (and automatically serves the whole as well).

As the great author-poet Thoreau wrote: *"If one advances confidently in the direction of his dreams, and endeavors to live the life which he has imagined, he will meet with success unexpected in common hours."*

Is it possible that all or most of the issues in the world are happening because humans are out of Balance? Is it possible we can return to Balance and create a New more rewarding-enlightened world (starting with ourselves, how we feel)? Is it possible that our relationship issues at home and at work are often because we are stressed, drained, and not feeling our best? Yes! It's time.

Note, as I state in my book, 'Path of the Enlightened Leader(s)' Energy, Wellness is so important because on a simple 1-10 scale: 1 being dead and 10 being alive, awake, and totally present – where do we need to be each day to feel good, and be effective at life? Where do you need to be each day to accomplish our mission? It's a win-win, for you and others when your energy is strong. Energy is the essential for all of our life.

In the following pages, we will lay out a template for a balanced living life plan which focuses on you, in the spirit of the research and teachings of the many experts and mentors we have learned from.

Are you ready to answer these Questions of life for you?
To become more aware?
To make different Choices?
To lead an energetically happier, more Balanced Life?

Still at lunch...

Sybrian: So, Mac. What do you think so far?

Mac: A lot of it sounds like stuff I've heard before, but I feel like there's more in just this one part I need to explore.

Sybrian: Like what?

Mac: Well, time management stuff....we talk about that all the time at the office. How to organize and prioritize tasks, but this isn't just about prioritizing my "to do" list. This is about taking the time to look at what's important, or priority, for me so I feel good about myself, what I'm spending my time on, and my life.

Sybrian: Go on....

Mac: It's about not always worrying about the "should do" or "have to" stuff. That's not living my life. It's fulfilling what someone else has decided for me, in a way. I've been struggling up the corporate ladder for years, haven't gotten as far as I wanted to....but then again.....

Sybrian: Then again....what?

Mac: I'm not sure that's actually what I want. Ever since I was a little kid, I watched my Dad work for his company and climb the ladder. He never really seemed all that happy, but we had plenty of money.
Growing up, we were all taught what success is supposed to be and what it is supposed to look like. And that is supposed to make us happy. I know it's not making me happy.

Sybrian: So, what next?

Mac: I need to take a look at why I'm doing what I do. Not just my job, but in my life. I feel like I'm missing out on something. But I'm really not sure where to go from here.

Sybrian: Let's get to creating your map to see where we need to explore next. Shall we?

Mac: Absolutely.

Boldness has Genius

"Until one is committed, there is hesitancy, the chance to draw back. Concerning all acts of initiative (and creation), there is one elementary truth, the ignorance of which kills countless ideas and splendid plans: that the moment one definitely commits oneself, then Providence moves too. All sorts of things occur to help one that would never otherwise have occurred. A whole stream of events, issues from the decision, raising in one's favor all manner of unforeseen incidents and meetings and material assistance, which no man could have dreamed would have come his way. Whatever you can do, or dream you can do, begin it. Boldness has genius, power, and magic in it. Begin it now."

- William Hutchinson Murray *(1913-1996),*
from his 1951 book entitled The Scottish Himalayan Expedition *– quoting Goethe couplet.*

Chapter 2: Balance

The topic of balance is an interesting one in our lives. What is balance really? What is it to you?

The chart below, gives us 8 focal points to a great life.

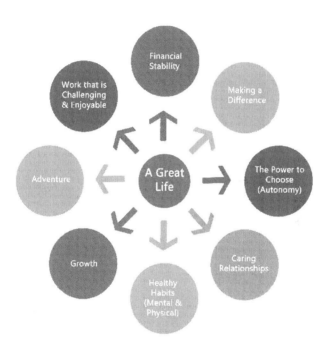

This implies that if we could juggle all of these in some particular formula we would be happy.

The challenge with this thinking is two-fold:

First, more than 80% of our waking life goes to work and we have just 4-6 left for living, eating, exercise, family, etc. That is the rub. There is a lot to do in a little amount of time! And it is vital to take care of you! So there is a lot more to this than simply pulling out a time management spread sheet and allocating hours to our tasks.

Second, with so little time, then, ask... what is your life Mindset, what are your priorities? This is the better question. Because once you know your top 3, everything else can pretty much melt away. It's a matter of simplification. You know? Every time management course I have ever taken, no matter how sophisticated eventually takes you to the point of deciding on priority. These time management tools can be very valuable for your many work tasks. Go to Franklin Covey, take their program, and get their planner. But before you do, let's explore your life, the bigger picture... what are *your* priorities?

To start, I ask you to fill in the pie chart (next page). Where does your time go?

This is to give you a clue of what is happening now. This may be your conscious priority; or it may not. This is a key point. For once you see it, you have the rest of the book to explore it and ask, is this what you want (choose)?

So take your time, take note, and reflect. Identify: What shifts or changes (decisions) are needed in your life now? At the end of the book, I'll ask you to do this same pie chart again. Just so you can see it.

The journey is... are you moved, can you see what's vitally important and what's changed? And how does this inner shift equate to a shift in time (choices)? Let's find out...

Priorities

Where does 'my time' go now?

Create categories and designate hours spent... (in the wheel below) using these or other elements:

Work	Self Time	Exercise
Family	Commuting	Sleeping
Service	Adventure	Learning
Spiritual	Socializing	Other

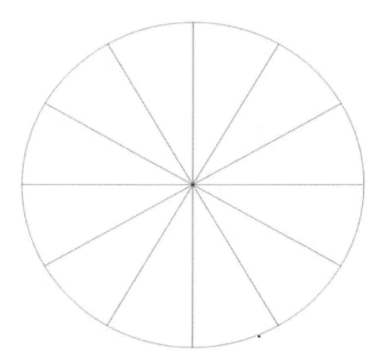

What does this wheel exercise tell you?
What new choices are calling?

Some thoughts that may help you on the path of Priority...

Three Keys to Magic –
From the Book, The Magicians Way, by William Whitecloud

Key One: Focus Creates Reality

What you focus on, you manifest. Like a golfer swinging a club, the ball tends to go where 'our mind is focused' when we swing. The Focus is critical, for the body/the universe will naturally find a way to complete the picture. Focus creates flow. Intention proceeds result.

What are your rituals, to consistently and passionately Focus on what you truly want? It won't happen by accident. Your focus should be the desired end result as 'here now'. What is your intention right this moment, your motive? What is your Focus? When you go astray simply reframe and return to Focus.

Imagination/dreaming are more powerful than 'reality'. A new dream, as in a new focused intention that you nourish each day, is the foundation to a new reality. Believe it, know it, feel it. Stay with it and... It appears.

Key Two: Thoughts and Feelings aren't Real: Or are they?

Your thoughts and feelings mean nothing more than telling you/giving you feedback on what you are focused on.

We all have feelings (emotions), I know I do, and this key was challenging for me to believe, for I Feel a lot! But if we're honest most feelings and emotions are reactions to our mind's focus. Learn from this and go back to your intended Focus.

With passionate Focus, you will be guided forward. Listen to your intuition (true feelings from your body, if you will), God talking to you, as to any steps to take.

How do you deal with emotion? Do you get emotional and distracted by your issues? Do your mind's fears, insecurities, and constant complaining about what's not here take away from your focus? If you have deep stuff going on, and we all do... find a professional healer-therapist to help you. Get yourself Free! Will you?

When you notice negative emotions, what can you do? Shift to silence, calm, and return to your Focus. Stop-Challenge-Choose (focus again). Ask God-Goddess for support. Follow His-Her promptings in your intuition.

Key Three: The Structure has integrity

All results come from a system (offering freedom within a framework). Buildings are created from an Architectural plan. Good cooking comes from a recipe and cooking process. The banks of a river support the flow of the river. Successful lives come from success rituals.

If something isn't working, go to the root and see what the structure is (and change it), or if there isn't one (create one), and fix it once and for all.

For example, if you keep losing your keys... knock a nail in the wall by the door and then systematically place them on the nail every time you enter the house. A structure - a home for the keys! Presto, issue solved. Are you using structures to help you?

There are more keys, of course, but these 3 are the foundation.

Keep these in mind as well:
- Everyone has a Heart
- Inspired action, not just 'doing'

- Hold the vision through it all
- Keep the energy Up
- It takes will
- Trust - Let it in...
- Learn the detailed 'skills' of magic; learn them and practice!

Get the book: The Magician's Way by William Whitecloud at Amazon.com.

Summary Questions:

How do these three keys (focus, emotions, structure) relate to taking care of yourself and to your life balance?

What do you *really*, *truly*, deep down inside, want?

Peace, joy, happiness, success, money? How do you get them?

What is the role of Energy or feeling good in getting them?

What do you make of the power of Choice to change your life, do you exercise it frequently?

If you don't have answers to these questions right now, it's okay! Let's explore some more...

Back at the Diner…

Mac: Wow….That's a lot for me to work with right there!

Sybrian: So, what are you going to do first?

Mac: I already worked out the Balance Chart. (He shows her a napkin with his pie chart.) When I look at where I'm spending most of my time, I can see it's really in the least important area I want to focus on. I've been not only working my regular hours, but I've been putting in a lot of extra time too…staying late, working weekends.

Sybrian: Are you working on a special project or have a pressing deadline?

Mac: Not really. I think I've just fallen into the trap of working more to try to get another promotion. I mean, the next level promotion means I won't have to travel so much, but I've been stuck for a long time where I am. When I look at how much time I'm spending at work without getting the results I want, and how little time I'm spending things I care about for me, I think I should look at making a change.

Sybrian: What kind of things did you enjoy doing that you're not doing now?

Mac: I used to enjoy gardening, building stuff, and having cookouts in the backyard, but I haven't done anything like that lately. I am starting to see why I'm feeling so dragged down and grumpy.

Sybrian: You are seeing the imbalances in your life.

Mac: Yeah.

Sybrian: So, what's your next step?

Mac: I've wanted to design a new garden area in the backyard. And my wife wants an addition to the deck. I think I'll start this weekend on that.

Sybrian: Today is Tuesday….why wait to get started? Can't you start working on your plans for the projects? Maybe talk to your wife at supper and get some ideas going?

Mac: I haven't been home for supper in weeks since I've been working late and on the road so much. Betty and I haven't been talking too much lately, much less doing or planning anything together. That's another place in my life that's out of balance.

Sybrian: So…what are you going to do about these imbalances?

Mac: I'm going to call my wife, ask her out to supper….like a date. And I'll ask her to help me get some ideas for the deck area. It'll give us a good place to start talking about something. You know, this already feels good!!

Sybrian: You'd better give her a call before someone else asks her out!

Mac: In a few minutes. There's something else.

Sybrian: What's that?

Mac: I noticed when I shifted my focus and energy to something I enjoy and something I can share with Betty, I started to feel better…without even trying!

Sybrian: Anything else?

Mac: Yeah, I think I need to create a new pattern, kind of like that key on a nail thing.

Sybrian: Like what kind of pattern?

Mac: I'm not sure yet. I can see where I need to change my thinking on a few things. I can see that I need to take better care of myself so I can take care of others.

Sybrian: Okay, anything else?

Mac: I think I need to feel like I can do things I enjoy for no other reason than I enjoy them. It's been so long since I've even thought about enjoying anything. I'm not sure what I want and I'm not too sure how to get there once I figure it out!

Sybrian: Well, you're in luck! The next part of our map is leading you right where you need to go to explore some of what you are talking about. How about you make that call to Betty?

Mac: I'm making the call and then, I want to discover more. Lead the way!

Sybrian: Actually, that 'guru' Bill is leading the way. You'll get some focus, fill up the positive energy, and when you let it flow out into the other parts of your life, you will start to really feel the difference!

Mac: Hey, it's working so far! I already feel energized!

Sybrian: So, are you ready?
Mac: Yep! I AM Ready!!

Sybrian: Step one: make that phone call! Now!

The Path

"When we study all the different religions, cultures, and human walks of life, we begin to see common traditions and customs that all people do to show honor in their own way. These are the common truths. All people have a form of prayer, a form of personal self-sacrifice, like fasting, or sun dancing, or some kind of vow. All people have some form of new birth like being baptized, or the sweat lodge ceremony. We all commune with the Holy Spirit in our own way. But we are all communing with the same Creator. God loves diversity. That is why Creator made us all different.

There is no one right or wrong way to worship God. The great Creator Spirit knows what is in our hearts. God likes it when we worship in our own way and when many people of different ways worship together sharing their ways. This greatly pleases Creator. There should be no judging, only a sharing of knowledge for understanding. It is time to see that we have much to learn from each other. The path of life is wide. There are many courses leading to the same destination. We all twist and turn, weaving our own course along the path of life. That is how we learn and grow.

If you were an investigator looking into a car accident and you only interviewed one witness, you would only have one account of the event. However, if you interviewed 14 people that saw the accident, you would have 14 different versions of the scene of events. You would see an overall true picture of what really happened.

The same is true with spirituality. But we cannot see the truth if we look with judgment based on what we believe to be true. We must be open to understanding. To love God is to love all of creation, including each other."

-Tim Walking Bear

Chapter 3: The Quest

"If you don't know your purpose, discover it, now. The core of your life is your purpose. Everything in your life, from your diet to your career, must be aligned with your purpose if you are to act with coherence and integrity in the world. If you know your purpose, your deepest desire, then the secret of success is to discipline your life so that you support your deepest purpose and minimize distractions and detours." - *David Deida*

The Native American Medicine Wheel
The medicine wheel is a Native American teaching... a spiritual guidance system to help us understand life through 4 stages of development.

Stage 1 the east is Vision.
Stage 2 the south is Challenge.
Stage 3 the west is Healing.
Stage 4 the north is Maturity.

We will use this model to guide us and to help us create our maps as we progress through various parts of the journey to a more balanced life.

Stage 1 (the East) is Vision:
Who am I? What do I want?
This suggests we need to be clear from our heart who we are and what we want. This is your unique expression of the real you; the you who is not living through the eyes or expectations of others.

Stage 2 (the South) is Challenge (Chaos):
How do I overcome the challenge of the three distracters? We pull out our warrior sword and cut out all the distraction, fears, and addictions that keep pulling us down.

Stage 3 (the West) is Healing:

Using Unity, Energy, Impeccability (the core process) to live more fully as your true self. This is practicing the healing path to live balanced lives.

Stage 4 (the North) is Maturity:

Mastering the daily path in a sustainable way. When we master our lives, we are happier more often than not and we are living and being our true selves.

Stage 1: Finding the Path: Higher Self/Lower Self

What do we want? Not an easy question. But we know more than we realize. We can start to understand ourselves, who we are, what we don't want, what we long for from our true self.

If we were to simplify the last 1000 years of psychology, philosophy and spiritual studies we may find that there are two parts of every human being seeking our attention: The Higher Self (HS) and Lower Self (LS).

To me, the 'path' is to understand and live more in our true self (HS) also known as Soul (our bodies and our bodies wisdom is connected to soul). Becoming more loving and wise and with this authentic power encourage our wonderful LS to take a supporting role. Simple really.

The higher self is our older, wiser, in the moment heart self. It is the seat of our soul where our wisdom, strength and compassion live. It is us, all of us, which is the uniqueness of 'me'. It is love. It is the part that says 'I am good enough!'

The LS is the baggage of our fear based ego minds. It is home to our wounds, the obsessive need for approval, control, security, our thoughts, wishes, fears, etc. that have been on a rampage to hurt and destroy our spirit, other people, and the planet. Have you noticed any of this in your life? LS is the 'not love' part of us. It is the part that says, "I am NOT good enough!" Fear rules him.

To understand this core principle of Self, for it may be new to you, simply refer to all paths of enlightenment: Zen meditation, Hindu Yoga, Sufi Poetry, Judeo-Christian Rites, Native American Ceremony. All of these are seeking that we rise; that we birth ourselves to our highest loving, and courageous, compassionate true self. This is cool. We all want the same thing: to be the highest love/Joy we can be.

Speaking Wind, used to say it's all about living as who we truly are. To dare to be our true self, which has nothing to do with our roles in life or others opinions, but with what our spirit is truly here to experience and express. He told me the place of the elders is Joy and that it would be the last frontier after we finally stopped chasing what no longer serves us. Will we discover and unleash this spirit within. The only question is... now or later?

> *"Remember that your natural state is joy."*
> *- Dr. Wayne W. Dyer*

Knowing we have these different Selves is one thing; living with wisdom (awareness and choice) is another. Knowing is good, it's a first step. Knowing helps understanding, while Wisdom (awareness and choice) is doing it. This is the tough part. We all talk about it, analyze it, and read about it. We ask the experts about it. When do we live it (our HS) and live it together as a global family?

This book is about how do we live in our True and unique HS so that love will guide us. From HS we make the choices that take us to the life we desire; From LS only to hurt and upset.

Why is this important you might ask? Look around. What do you see? Have we created a world of peace, love, courage and understanding (HS) or one of dog eat dog competition, fear, stress, and violence (LS)?

When we look deep into ourselves, it is even more telling. Ask, how many times per day do you live in the past or future versus the present? Love versus fear? Can you see how comical this is?

We almost never live in the now. Now is where the HS lives. The HS is our heart that talks to us in stillness. All else is noise from our LS minds trying to repeat the insanity of the past and take it into the future.

The LS seeks but will not find. It tests us by going into places that will bring us back to 'not good enough'. This is not to say that the LS is bad; nor is the mind, memory, experience, skill, brains, or even the shadow. All is helpful. The question is, is this truly you?

The answer is no. LS is the machinery of you. You are not this. You are HS: Pure spirit, pure witness. LS is our drama based 'personality' which deserves our love when it so requires, which is always. See it as a wounded child needing our love. Never fight or try to destroy your LS. The key is to get it (him, her) to work with us. When it takes over, we are a mess. It's about choosing which consciousness we will abide by.

For example, there is nothing wrong with a healthy dose of sexual attraction (even if you're in a marriage or relationship); it happens, it's normal, this is a part of each of us, we get attracted to people. In the consciousness of HS, we handle this with honor, love, truth, a sense of fun, and sacredness. We smile as we maintain our boundaries and keep on dancing together as one.

In the consciousness of the LS, we may chase after, cheat, use others, become addicted, hurt each other, and become obsessed. It is never the subject, but rather the consciousness in which we approach it.

Take another challenging topic like killing another living thing. People say all the time, "I would never kill anything". Yet each day, even those of us who are vegetarians, we kill repeatedly believe it or not, whether it is for food to eat, microorganisms in and around our being, or just going for a walk a stepping on insects we may not see. For others there is hunting, fishing, soldiering…you name it. The question is not whether we will kill in life, it is will we be conscious about it?

This all sounds very eastern or Buddhist, hence folks often ask me, 'What is your religion Bill? Are you a Christian or, are you a Buddhist?' Does the answer really matter?

I say, I seek what is true in each of the world's teachings. I have learned from them all and share what I have learned with you; Call it whatever turns you on. I call it waking up, being conscious…Conscious, meaning being aware. What am I doing? Where am I coming from (HS, LS; Love or fear), etc.?

The Dalai Lama stated it best, "My religion is compassion, and I have no other." Love is everything. Love is what Jesus, all great teachers, and saints have shown us.

In physical form however, love can seem quite complex. What exactly is love? I am not talking about romance, or enabling, or giving yourself away or any of that. It is about us…me, you, each individual… living from a foundation of love and being that love.

I see this love, in its essence, as **Acceptance and Creation.**

Back at the Diner... a couple of days later....

Sybrian: Hey, Mac! How was dinner the other night?

Mac: You know, it was a great night. I took Betty out to dinner. When I started talking to her about redoing the deck, at first, she didn't believe me! She said I was gone so much that I probably didn't have the time. I told her I was going to reprioritize how I've been spending my time. She was still skeptical. At first, it started to bring me down.

Sybrian: So, how did you get past that? You said it was a great night.

Mac: It was probably the best time we've had together in a long time. Anyway, I just asked her to humor me and she did. The more we talked, the more excited she became with it.

She had some great ideas and we were drawing plans out on the napkins until the place was ready to shut down! We were having fun together. It was nice to hear her laugh. This energy stuff must be contagious!

Sybrian: (laughing) Yes, it is. I'm glad you had a good time. Did you get through any more of the book?

Mac: I've been reading this stuff, but I'm a little confused on some of it.

Sybrian: Like what?

Mac: All my life, everyone told me the opposite of love was hate. It's not?

Sybrian: No, it isn't. The base emotion hate stems from is fear. Your Lower Self operates more from a fear base; your Higher Self operates from a love base. You want your Higher Self, or HS to be predominate or "in charge", if you will.

Mac: Lower Self and Higher Self? So the opposite of Love is...Fear?

Sybrian: Yes.

Mac: This is starting to make sense to me. We can't just get rid of our LS?

Sybrian: No, we can't. It's a part of us. It has a job to do. It is where our experience lies. LS is part of our self-protection. It's essential. We have to learn how to work with our LS and not let the negative parts of it take control.

Our higher, more authentic selves come from the HS. If we only had HS, we'd give instead of share and that would deplete us to the point of no longer having anything to give. But acting from the LS base is acting, and being, out of the fear and hurt of our past. We need both the LS and the HS because together they are part of our balance of being.

Mac: So, we have to make the LS and the HS work together?

Sybrian: Yes. It is part of the balance.

Mac: What is this about love being Acceptance and Creation? I'm not sure I'm getting this exactly.

Sybrian: Well, seeing where you left off, that's the next part. Bill explains this very well, but a lot of times, it helps to have someone to talk over the concepts with, especially if they are new to you. So, let's read this part now.

Mac: Let's do it!

Acceptance and Creation

Acceptance (non-doing) means Being present, letting go, surrendering, and being authentically with whatever is. If someone is in fear (including us), the antidote is love.

As a first step, even if for a few moments, start to slow down and enjoy more silence, affirming that all is divine order, even with our (or the worlds) imperfections. Right here, right now, with my mind quieted, all is truly perfect as it is. There is nothing needed in this moment. God-Goddess, Great Spirit is in charge and all is well. Only my wandering judgmental LS mind causes me hell. So, I accept it all, let go, relax; there is nowhere to go, nothing to do right now! How freeing. Just stop. Unplug. Be Peace. Be HS.

Hence, simply trust and affirm that the highest outcome is happening naturally. Even within the deepest moment of despair, know that you are greater than your despair or circumstances. You are cared for by the divine. You can stop, undo, be, and wait. Acceptance asks us to find the beauty in non-doing, by being gentle and peaceful with yourself, with all beings, and with all relations.

Creation (doing) is inspired, birthed from this HS place of acceptance, of gentleness, of self-love, the nonviolence at the root of all religions. This means that as we slow down, listen to our true heart, see what it asks of us, then we are clear and can lovingly, courageously, and diligently act with simplification, precision and love.

We are given many visions from our heart, mind, and soul. We are to bring those visions to life, to enjoy, to better the world around us through our businesses, projects, foundations, etc. Because our visions are what we are, it is our passion to go out and do it. So listen to you!

Hear the need to take better care of yourself, to eat right, live with honor, enjoy each moment and, just do it. Listen to the voice deep within your being that tells you, encourages you to dance more, to have fun, to smile, and to love. Then do all you can each day to serve these heart visions.

You are like a master gardener who plants the seed. Then each day you go out to your garden to water and till the garden to help it grow. Of course, we don't make it grow; the sun, soil, rain does it. We support with our doing.

So listen to your heart and till your garden. This is the path of love. This is true spirit discipline. Mastering ourselves is the ultimate mastery. The mastery of self-love and the love for our creations that Great Spirit is expressing through us is our Higher Self.

> *"Do you know what you are?*
> *You are a manuscript of a divine letter. You are a*
> *mirror reflecting a noble face.*
> *This universe is not outside of you. Look inside*
> *yourself;*
> *Everything that you want, you are already that."*
>
> *- Rumi*

One of my teachers from San Diego, a gentleman from India, summed up the path this way:

"Be Quiet (be still) each day and go to Satsang (group meditation community) each week. Meditation and similar practices are a way of 'being still' so you can unravel from your mind and the beliefs that were taught to you that you have never reviewed to see if they are worth following."

Satsang is a forum where we can gather together and reflect on life with others on the same path. This book is a form of Satsang ... a humble guide, with a Life plan with daily, weekly, monthly and quarterly adherences to get you started on your chosen way.

Once you're on your way, find 'Satsang' helpers/

community in your local area in which to share. This is foundational to the 'Walk in Balance' path to health, wellness, and mastery, to be who you are, happy, no matter what our circumstances. Be quiet, go to Satsang.

And note, that this is an inner game (with support of course). For is God 'out there'? Is God/Great Spirit a Santa Claus or a baby sitter sitting on a cloud? I see too many of us run to the parish priest, the shaman, and the psychics of the world every time we have an issue, or decision. This reinforces that they are knowledgeable, and we are not. This is not true.

We all need help and mentoring time to time, but only we can make the choices for our own lives. For in each of our hearts is the exact DNA of the Great Spirit, residing there inside of you. Did you know this? This is not to say, that we cannot learn from others, get support, or pray to God or Spirit helpers in your own words for help. Of course pray! It simply means that we must listen to ourselves, to our own heart!

As it says in the opening to the Gospel of St Thomas, "The Kingdom of God is within... it is in no church or building". Ask rarely advice from others, get quiet and ask your own heart, because therein lie the answers directly from God; The God, in you; The Spark of Him/Her, HE/SHE that lives <u>within</u> you. Only then do we understand who we really are.

Let us no longer be slaves to all the supposed holy ones, or to our parent's beliefs (as truth without exploration), or to all others' opinions of what and who we are to be. In my view, it is healthy to realize, "we are the holy one." We are the ones we have been waiting for; the one we must live with. The only teachers I have respected were the ones who told me to go inside and to trust myself-the God within me (in me and in all); this is a great truth!

The Path of Acceptance and Creation is one of love.
It is discovering your True Self.
It is living fully as this Self...
Learning, healing, loving, serving, and playing in Joy.

Remember this is deep work and requires daily practice, yet it isn't drudgery. It's simply nourishment, fun, and playful! It's fun to learn, to grow, and to love. It's fun to be our best, and commune with like-minded people practicing the same. Enjoy the gift of celebrating effective living! Make everything a pleasure! Embrace the pain, embrace the Joy. Now is the time to live!

The key here is a Life Plan (Map), with our intents to organize our practice of acceptance and creation. Daily, weekly, monthly, and quarterly adherence will help us to stay in our hearts and live healthy. Again, this is not a required list of 'have to's'.

These are gifts, recommendations I offer that you can choose to do or not, or make up your own. It's up to you.

Let us begin your Map.

Exercises:

They are simple and easy, so just have fun with them.

Turn the page ...

Uh-Oh… Resistance at the Diner……

Mac: I'm not going to do the exercises. So, let's keep reading.

Sybrian: Umm….that's not really a good idea to skip the exercises.

Mac: Why is that?

Sybrian: The exercises are an important part of taking the steps, of finding out where you are now, and where you want to go.

Mac: I know what I want. It's all in my mind and I got it.

Sybrian: No. That's not how this works.
Do you know that I have found, when a person won't take the first step, it's guaranteed that they won't take any of the next ones?

By writing down your intentions, journaling, and the rest, it helps create the positive, joyful energy you are going to need to make the rest of your journey.
Doing these exercises is the first step!

Mac: So, I have to write this stuff down?

Sybrian: Yes. Remember how good you felt when you shared the garden and deck idea with Betty?

Mac: Yes.

Sybrian: And what did you and Betty do all through supper?

Mac: We drew up plans and ideas for the garden.

Sybrian: You drew them up? You mean, you wrote them down *on a bunch of napkins, right?*

Mac: Well, yes. We wrote them down and drew diagrams of the garden project so we would know what we need to do to make the garden and deck how we want them. So?

Sybrian: This is EXACTLY like that! You have to write it down, make your plans, create your steps...so you know what you need to do to get what you want. But in this case, it's for your life, not just your backyard garden!

Mac: Oh....I see!! I get it! Okay, let's do this thing!

Sybrian: Here's a notebook I got for you. No more napkins.

Mac: A notebook. You mean, my "journey journal"?

Sybrian: Pretty much.

Mac: Okay, exercises....writing things down...here I come....

Sybrian: But not here in the diner. How about you work on this and I'll meet you Sunday afternoon?

Mac: Sounds good. Hey, why don't you come by the house to see what we've gotten done outside? Betty would love to see you again.

Sybrian: Great! See you then!

Exercises:

Please do not move on until you do these exercises.

I know a lot of people bog down over "what to write" and others decide "I don't need to do this or write it down". Doing the exercises and writing is part of your commitment to your Journey and to make Walk in Balance work for you. You are creating your map for the path you choose to follow. Short cutting is the longer route. These answers are only for you, so relax, play, and have fun.

Exercise 1:
What do you…from your Higher Self…..really want?

This is a question where people either struggle or know instantly what the answers are.

Simply pray in the language of your own heart to whom you love to pray for guidance and enter into the silence of being with yourself (and your Spirit helpers). You can meditate, go for a long walk in the woods or on a beach, sit by a stream or campfire… wherever you can be quiet. You may decide to do a Journey Process where you ask your Higher Self (heart) for a response. You will get one, for it is there. There is no wrong answer. Write everything down that comes to you whether it seems relevant or not; whether it seems realistic or not. This is your Vision Quest!

To give you a little insight as to what a Journey Process is, here is an excerpt from Way of the Corporate Shaman: "In some ways, a Journey is like a guided meditation. It's really nothing esoteric or unusual. If you ever visualize or dream, you already Journey. You don't need special intuitive abilities or a lot of training. It is a quite simple process, and most "get it" the first time. In my experience, it helps to work with a healer who uses a drum. The drum acts as a gentle aid to deepen our awareness state. Its slow, monotonous beat lulls the conscious mind to rest (become itself to visit realms rich in archetypal symbolism born of human earthly experience spanning many millennia." Note: If you are interested in reading more from <u>Way of the Corporate Shaman</u>, it is available through most online book sources.

For those of you who want help, I can guide you through this individually in a Shift coaching session. See end of the book for more.

Either way, once you begin your Silence or Journey, you will use the pages ahead to answer from the heart:

What do you...from your Higher Self.....really want?
Who am I? (I AM beauty, joy, love, God, courage, etc.)
What do I choose? (From your HS, your heart core)

Just write...free flow until it's done!

What do I really want ...

What do I really want …

Reflection:
As you listen to your heart, look at what you have written.
Reflect.
What do you notice?

Is the list about giving, getting, or experiencing life?
What else do you notice?
What does this tell you about yourself?

Once you are done, move on to the path of intention and action. Intention means to reduce down your wants to the core of what it is you are specifically after.
Better yet, what is after you!

Turn page…

Exercise 2: Turn the vision into three core heart desires.
Test them by asking, "What does this **truly** give me?"
Get to the core! Do this now! Ask, FEEL, see what core
desires have the most Life for you, Circle your top 3.

**What are my top three priorities/intentions for my life
right now** in order to be able to "Walk in Balance"? (Be as
specific as possible. Ex: Be happy-healthy; having loving
relationships; create 3 new happy clients at work, etc.)
(note: Just writing them down begins birthing them)

1

2

3

How will I nourish these desires? What specific daily
actions will you take to support each of your three
priorities? This is your "doing" part.

Nourish

1

2

3

What makes these three items a priority for me? (This is
your "WHY do it?") WHY you do something is important to
keep in mind. It is your fuel for your actions towards your
intentions.

Why is this intent so Important to me?

1

2

3

My Three Intentions/ Nourishing Actions/ Why CHART

Summarize here -

Intention	Nourish Action	Why
1		
2		
3		

Exercise 3:

Take a few moments and write a Walk in Balance Mission Statement for your life.

A mission statement is a way to identify your key mission, or dream for how you want to live your life. To discover your life mission, simply ask yourself the main question, "What drives me on a soul-spirit level, if money and circumstances were no issue?"

You can also ask yourself questions such as: What do I enjoy? What do I want for my life? How do I want to live? What do I stand for? Take some time where you can be by yourself to find your true HS answers. These are the answers which live in your heart; they are your deepest sense of meaning and your deepest desires. Reflect on what you know, want, and love.

Example (to borrow from):

My dream is to be happy and to slow my life down and play, to know myself, grow in maturity, and share my gifts. My greatest gift is living my natural genius of _____; as I share my genius I Feel JOY and I fulfill my mission. My foundation for living is comprised of the following principles: _____, _____, and _____. I live a life of _____by learning, loving, and sharing_____ so I can experience _____. IAM _____ _____ _____ _____.

Dream Journal... (ideas)
*(*No need to be perfect, it's an exploration!)

My Walk in Balance Mission Statement – Dream:
Trust the words that flow

Let's reflect for a moment. If you went deep within yourself, can you see how much substance there is in what you wrote? Did you discover things which surprised you, about how important personal well-being/experiencing life is to you? And/or the personal well-being of those you love? More and more people are focusing on core heart values rather than lists of material items. This says something very important in our culture – that more and more are awakening to something deeper. And, if you are clear in your heart that the new home, a new car, an affluent job is key to your path right now...go after it! You choose. Otherwise, embrace the truest urgings that your heart calls for and Enjoy your vacation time here on earth.

Maybe that's all this is, life: a time to love and a time to enjoy the journey of the lessons we are here to experience. Whatever happens, laugh, for some things work out and some do not. Just be with it. As a great teacher once said, ***If it comes, let it come... if it goes, let it go***. Do your best, whatever happens, detach, learn, and trust. It is all for a good reason. Or you can overdo and die young of a heart attack, I've seen it, I bet you have too. **Remember, this is a HS path, not the ego LS path.** This is not about goals and hard work per se. It's about intention and nourishment, being your joyful self, and with joy as your compass... create what you need for you and yours. It's a balanced pathway to happiness and fulfillment.

Author, Stephen Cope, says it this way:
"Find your true self (HS) and what your HS loves to do (intention). Live from there; give all your passion (nourishment) to living this self fully. Let go of the fruits of your pursuits. Whatever happens, let it be, we cannot control it. Give it all to God. Do it out of devotion to God and for the sheer joy of expressing it – which are one in the same! (Of course, use common sense, make a good living, and be prosperous in a healthy way that works for you.)"

The focus is the joy revolution... it is about feeling good!! And when we feel good, we reclaim our power, everything flows, and we mostly don't really care about all the stuff anymore, you know? Most of us want stuff to feel good, did you know that... why not feel good first! And then if you want stuff, it's all for fun, eh? It's a playful game.

Creating the Map Exercise

This is where you will use the exercises used so far to complete your personal Walk in Balance Map. It's very simple. Your Mission-Intentions are your destination. Where you are now is your starting point. Everything in between (supporting actions) is your journey.

Now I am going to remind you about the Three Keys to Magic. Remember those? They are: Focus, Thoughts and Emotions, and Structure.

Your Map will help you keep your focus directed towards your priorities and intentions (in the spirit of 'already done'). Thoughts and emotions help fuel your actions in support. Structure creates the freedom within a framework, a foundation of the steps of your journey, aka your Map.

No matter what your intentions are, focusing on them (visualizing them happening, being grateful for etc.) should make you feel good. This will raise your vibrational energy and help create the thoughts and emotions (energy) to motivate your actions. Structure helps guide which actions to do next.

Of course, you will have to commit yourself to your Walk in Balance Map. This means read it often, take the daily actions listed and of various sorts to create what you want to create, do what you want to do, live how you want to live, and be the person you want to be. Turn the page …

My Walk in Balance Life MAP (initial draft)
(Fill In below...)

Name _____   **Date** _____

I.   My Mission – Dream is:

II.   Intentions

Intention	Nourish Action	Why
1		
2		
3		

III.   _My_ Daily Walk in Balance Wellness Practices, to support me in feeling energized and great (no matter what): _(to come from the rest of this book...)_

42

(Suggestions for **III.** for now...)

- Meditate and pray each morning.
- Read your Life Map and follow it, affirm it.
- Exercise/Movement (walk, bike, swim, yoga) minimum ___ minutes per day. Smile.
- Journal on your successes and key learnings, then meditate before bed.
- Stay soul connected in weekly spiritual groups. (ongoing)

So there you have it, a wonderful first draft of your map on who you are, what you want, and what you will do for it (a final draft for you to fill out will be in the chapter 6, so gather and prepare for that).

With the Map...

There is an old saying where the attention goes, the energy flows. Having this map gives you power... the power of intention and the power of choice. You now have a Life Focus, a request if you will to give the universe to bless and for you to nourish (co-creation of your Walk in Balance).

Let us continue, there is so much more fun to explore ...

Sunday afternoon… in the garden…

Mac: Well, what do you think?

Sybrian: Wow…this is great! And you're starting to look like you're a little happier too.

Mac: It feels really good to be working on this with Betty. We worked all day and it was probably the best couple of days we've had together in a long time. We dug in the dirt, laughed, and had fun.

Sybrian: A couple of days?

Mac: Yep. I took a personal day on Friday.

Sybrian: That's awesome! I love those flower boxes. I've never seen anything like them.

Mac: Betty designed them and I made them.

Sybrian: Super creative!

Mac: We made a good team on this project. And it was fun.

Sybrian: Mac, I can see your excitement, but I'm also feeling like there's something else. Is there something bothering you?

Mac: Sort of. I mean, I am excited Betty and I had such a good time on this project. It definitely addressed my priority of improving my relationship with her.

Sybrian: But…

Mac: But when I was saying I wanted to do a garden project, I didn't mean I wanted to build flower boxes.

Sybrian: Didn't the two of you plan this together when you went out to eat last week?

Mac: Well, yes. But...you know, just let me show you what it was I had in mind.

Sybrian: Okay.
<They walk towards the back of the yard.>

Mac: I just started on this, but I'm creating a very special space. This is what I really wanted to work on when I said I wanted to do a garden project. I'm working on this by myself. I don't want Betty to see this until it's done.

Sybrian: This looks like a great place to make a quiet spot to read or meditate.

Mac: A long time ago, I planted this ring of shrubs around the oak trees. Betty is more interested in the deck area and flower beds you can see from the house, so I've worked on that first with her and I did enjoy doing it. This morning, I cleared this area.

Sybrian: What are you thinking of putting here?

Mac: I'm going to put in a small fish pond, maybe with a waterfall or fountain, and a small fire pit. Reading, meditating, and just having a quiet space in nature is what I'm going to create. I haven't finished planning it yet. I'll have to invite you back once it's done.

Sybrian: I'd like that. Now, where are you at with your Walk in Balance progress?

Mac: Here's what I've come up with so far. You were right about writing everything down. Once I did the exercises and started working on a few of the steps, I found I had more ideas I was really excited about.

Sybrian: That's great! So, where are you at now?

Mac: Well, the exercises were helpful, but I feel like there are parts missing from my map.

Sybrian: Like what?

Mac: I've got the "What I want". I've got the Creation (doing) part. I have my reasons "Why". I wrote my Mission Statement. I've been meditating, praying, taking steps, and writing in my journal.

Sybrian: Okay, so what's missing?

Mac: I keep finding myself having doubts and I'm not really sure exactly HOW I'm supposed to get to what I want. I've already hit a few obstacles and I'm not finding a way to get past them.

Sybrian: Like what?

Mac: I'm not sure about spending the money on the garden project.
I mean, I can afford to do it, but I'm not sure if I should.

Sybrian: Hmm....how about we go through the next couple of sections of the book now? I think some of your questions might be answered pretty easily.

Mac: Okay....let's go back up to the deck.

Law of Attraction

There has been a lot written about the Law of Attraction (LoA), as the principle of all life to get what we want. The LoA is the idea that we manifest/attract what/where we are (akin to karma). We are attractors by our thoughts.

The LOA has become the ultimate 'technique' espoused by many teachers as the key to life, the path for people to finally get what they want. But has our spiritual path ever been about getting stuff? Have you met people with all the stuff in the world, get whatever they want and they are miserable? What is the key?

To me, the key is about feeling better, being in and living from my Higher Self. I have learned being in the HS is the key to all life. The HS is where Acceptance and Creation meet, where love prevails and attraction ignites.

The LOA works when we are in our HS, because we are in our true light, happy, and magically alive, everything flows much better to us. This is mainly because we have lightened up. We are ok whether we get 'it' (the money, relationship, house, etc.) or not. We know we are happy.

The Law of Attraction does exist and it does work. "Ask, believe, receive" does exist. But, most people will not take the extra, unspoken step. Part of believing, is doing. This is because life is not about sitting on your couch eating bonbons and watching television all day waiting for the FedEx guy to deliver your package to you. Lol. Life is meant to be lived; not watched or waited for. Unless that works for you! Consider Taking very simple inspired actions, with belief and faith is a big part of LoA – and great fun too.

As you are doing, you create the higher vibrational energy required for LoA to work. Action also creates Joy. Joy creates attraction. And notice, whom do you find yourself attracted to...who shines in life? Those with a joyful being!

To be happy, follow the practices in this book and get alert to where you are each day on what I call the vibrational scale. Whenever you are below Joy, see it as a chance to rest, reflect and choose again. For ultimately, while all states are fine, only where Joy exists does man evolve.

Non-joy is the messenger to shift something.
Shift vibration!

Vibration scale
10. Joy!!! (Love and Above)
-

-

5. Okay...not happy, not sad
-

-

0. Depressed, lethargic, numb

So.... where do you want to be? Where does life work for you?

The soul is on a journey. There will be ups and down in life which we cannot control. Life will be life. There will be sickness, and down days; we succeed, we fail; there is loss and sadness. Yes.

By no means am I joyful each day. I often have to do things I don't 'love'...to pay the bills etc. Some things are pretty practical, 'chop wood carry water' activities. What I attempt to do is my best... to be present, to learn, to share where I can, and maybe even laugh at the wild ride that is life. Joy is the anchor to walking this path.

This being said, have you ever felt that happy go lucky feeling, that life is grand, that everything is going your way?

It's a wonderful feeling, yes? Yes! Is it possible to have this more often? To feel more consistently, our own true self, to feel this 'happy go lucky' joy! I bet each of us can.

The ultimate paradox of life is when we feel good we do not give much thought about what we think we need because we are relaxed, free and happy. Our real need(s) are met! When we feel great, all is well and it flows. When we feel great, we contribute positively to society, our families, to all around us. When we are down, that simply draws less to us so that we can <u>be</u> for a while. It means we need to re-center ourselves and find our balance.

The bottom line is that HS gives it all to us, feeling good and magnetizing our intentions. When you can enter the HS zone more and more and all will be given! This is a paraphrase of Saint Mark, "Seek first the Kingdom of God, and all things will be added unto you." How does that sound to you?

May I suggest we Walk in Balance by embracing the daily art of living in HS (acceptance). Give ourselves adequate time to be, to read our intentions (staying thought positive) and nourish them with daily loving action. (And of course, take care of the many daily chop wood and carry water parts of our life).

We simply trust the lion's share of life is God's doing and we do our small part by asking what our intentions need from us so we can nourish them to help them come to life. Remember the master gardener analogy. We love and nourish our garden (watering, tilling) while the universe is the one that 'grows it' together we shine and the garden flourishes. This is the miracle of God. It's all working out.

Steps to raise your vibrational energy:

Feel Great (Live in HS, Raise your Vibration through wellness)
X
Affirm Intentions, see as already here! (Visualize, Focused Thought Management—stay positive in faith)
X
Nourish intentions with your best love, gratitude and service - act where called and then let go/trust...

= Miracles Flow

If we do not know what we truly want... even just the essence... we can flounder in misery until we decide. But do not fear God is with us, guiding us.

So let this be play. Just do your best... deep down inside, I want to _____!!! I want to be happy, to Live, to enjoy, and make a difference! Whatever it is, write it down!!

Scream it, dance it, roar, laugh, be serious with it or life can pass by quickly and we can miss so much of it.

NOW is the time to ignite the flame within! Allow acceptance and creation to birth. Your heart is asking something of you... what is it?
The Universe is on your side... Place your order, move forward!

Ask, Believe, Receive.

Sybrian and Mac...

Mac: I don't "get" this Law of Attraction stuff. I've always believed that you work hard and get what you earn. It's always been at the top of my "Mumbo Jumbo" list as total hogwash.

Sybrian: Okay, anything else?

Mac: I keep finding myself having doubts and I'm not really sure exactly HOW I'm supposed to get to what I want without spending a lot of money.

Sybrian: Okay, those two things actually fit together. They are part of the puzzle pieces a lot of people miss towards living a more balance life. You've taken the first steps, which is great. You've hit the second stage of the Medicine Wheel: challenge (chaos).

Mac: Okay, and?

Sybrian: We'll start with the Law of Attraction. Have you ever noticed that when you are in a good mood and smiling, it seems that the people around you tend to be friendlier and more helpful?

Mac: Well....yes.

Sybrian: And when you are in a bad mood, people seem to be less than helpful, you run into more obstacles, and things in general just seem to go all wrong?

Mac: Yup. That seems to be the way things go.

Sybrian: In a very simple way, that is the Law of Attraction at work in your life. It's working all the time whether you know it or not.

When you are in a positive, good mood, people are helpful and friendly, things seem to go smoothly, and you overcome most obstacles with ease.

When you are in a negative bad mood, you are going to attract negative and "bad" things to you. Does that make sense?

Mac: It does for that. But what about all this "wealth attraction" so many of the "gurus" talk about?

Sybrian: Are you ready for this? It's more about making profits rather than being prophets. The "Ask, Believe, Receive" routine works best if you're building momentum towards it through your daily practices AND taking positive action. You have to be doing something positive for LoA to work for you, not be a lump on a log. And of course sometimes I just ask and it happens!

Mac: (laughing) Now, you're sounding like me!

Sybrian: Sort of. If you recall, Bill said that the LoA isn't about money, although that is often a side effect. You can have tons of money and be the most miserable person in the world, right?

Mac: Right. Since LoA is working all the time, we are attracting the good stuff AND the bad stuff.

Sybrian: Exactly!

Mac: But I don't want the bad stuff!

Sybrian: No one does, but when the "bad" things happen, that is where we grow and learn. Overcoming these things is part of the course of being human.

If you want the LoA to bring you the "good stuff", you have to consciously put forth those types of energy and thoughts. Walking in Balance is about living from your Higher Self, which activates the positive LoA.

Once you are able to do that, it will start bringing positive people and experiences into your life, which makes your LIFE richer and fuller than it was before. Obstacles and challenges are part of the balance. Joy and Love are other parts. Money is another part of the Balance.

Mac: Easy money is what those "gurus" all seem to focus on, even though now I'm seeing it's really not like that at all. How does having positive thoughts and energy make money?

Sybrian: But it's still not about the money. It's about living a loving and joyful life. Money is part of the equation because you need it to pay for things you need and want. You are raising your vibrational energy to attract "the good stuff" with the Law of Attraction.

Don't you notice that you tend to have more opportunities open to you when you are more positive? People and things are attracted to joy, love, happiness, friendliness, optimism, caring, and so forth. When you are operating from a negative plane or vibrational energy, doors tend to close rather than open.

It's all about raising your vibrational energy to match what you want to attract.

Mac: So, I should do the exercise Bill outlines to help raise my vibrational frequency as part of my daily practices?

Sybrian: Yep. That's why he put it there.

Mac: Okay, that answers the part about the Law of Attraction. Now, what about all the doubts and fears I'm having about HOW I'm going to get what I want? I still don't understand that part, because if I'm having fears and doubts, I'm not going to attract what I want. Right?

Sybrian: Let's go back to the book. There are three key items Bill will cover: Primary Distracters, Control Dramas, and Obstacles. Let me know if you want to stop for a discussion at any point, okay?

Mac: Okay, let's do it!

Chapter 4: The Challenge

Are we out of our Minds yet?

The path of HS is an awesome one, and luckily, our creator made it quite challenging with tests to see if we are serious about being happy! Ever been tested? Do we REALLY want to be our true self, to live in love, joy… in acceptance and creation? Or do we prefer drama?

The universe is always asking you, "Will you be you?" It's important that you know HS is not some perfect puritanical state. We are allowed to enjoy all sides of life: to sometimes be the poor confused 'two leggeds' that we are; and at other times to be divine… to enjoy life, and even indulge in that yummy dark chocolate you have had your eye on. Enjoy it. All is ok! Just do not eat the whole store out today, right? The key is to do what you do from heart (HS) and not from addiction (LS). Let's explore….

The Medicine Wheel teachings, stated in Stage 2, there are three distracters that we will explore in this chapter.

Stage 1 is Vision: What do you want?

Stage 2 is Chaos: How do I overcome the Challenge of the three distracters (addiction to approval, control, security).

The path to healing and maturity (HS) and to live a joyful life is to overcome the tests, which are the three primary distracters of (LS) in Stage 2. The distracters are cunning. They will test each of us in a different way every day. Be alert! That is what makes life such an interesting game.

We seem to be seeking love and happiness and all the while something else is seeking to test our commitment. It takes courage to love and be happy. Love is not some soft notion of caring alone. The heart is the place of courage, strength and honor as well as fun, joy and happiness! You may ask each day how may you be your higher self to love all of your complex tendencies, to overcome the distracters, and fulfill your heart's mission.

The Primary Distracters

The three primary distracters are all addictions to fear based thoughts, feelings, and behaviors. They are the addiction to approval, the addiction to control, and the addiction to security.

Primary Distracter 1: Seeking Approval (Outside vs In).

This is an interesting and ever pervasive issue in our world. Simply stated, this means that we are putting our energy out *there;* wanting the world or others to take care of us and tell us what to do etc. to make us feel happy.

This is a game of chasing our own tail, because we are living through another's eyes. Trying to be good, make the grade, and to be accepted.

The problem is there is no one who can truly make us feel good about ourselves (even if they tried). And, we can never be such great manipulators (aloof, poor me, victim...control dramas we will get to in a minute) that the world does what we want or approves of us.

We start seeking approval from others when we are very young. We are actually programmed and conditioned to seek the approval of our parents, teachers, and society at a very young age.

To prevent us from this past habit of being at the effect of things, as an adult, we let go and fulfill ourselves inwardly by following our own path and allowing ourselves to be who we are. To be strong so nothing may disturb our peace of mind. To be the master of our own lives.

We know who we are, we love ourselves, and we trust our own council (and of course we have friends and family who love us and support us, but we lead our lives, we approve of ourselves). Paradoxically when we do this... the universe and others do give us more. We must claim our own power. It begins with us!

Note: *"It is not what happens; it is what we do with what is that makes the difference. I am the master of my thoughts, feelings, and emotions. Through my path of self-love all else loves me too (and those who do not, I do not care)."*

Primary Distracter 2: Controlling (Trying to Force an Outcome).

If our attempts to manipulate the world passively do not work by doing what "they" want in order to gain approval, then we can seek to aggressively control (intimidator, interrogator ... control dramas), so that we do not feel as vulnerable to our mortality. The fact is no matter how smart we are; we are not in control of the world or what will happen.

This control shows up as too much work, force, push, and yang energy. Have you ever pushed? Doesn't it all stress you out, and it still never will go as planned? We eventually learn to do what we can, do our best, then trust and let go. We know all we can control is our own thoughts and deeds. We can control our responses to life through the adherence to our path; the rest is in God's hands. When we live from our HS with acceptance and creation, we win. We have peace and a greater likelihood that what we want will manifest because there is ease.

Planning and taking action (Life Map for example) is not the same as controlling; these can be helpful and are part of moving forward with our choices, to Walk in Balance.

So relax, maybe work less, and see how the world works perfectly without our policing or fixing it. Rather, trust. Intend, nourish, let go and affirm, allowing what will be will be.

Note: *"Let go and let God. We are in control of nothing but our actions/interpretations (thoughts, feelings, and emotions.) By listening to our hearts, God speaks and we know what is needed for happiness. We gently give what is needed and we receive the gift of expressing our true self, which is joyful no matter what the outcome."*

Primary Distracter 3: Seeking Security (In the past and future).

This is the subtlest and cunning distracter because we live in our over thinking heads and LS so much of the time (and we're not aware of it!). We find security in this familiar thinking which is always about the known of the past or in the projection of an idealized future (often both are filled with worry and anxiety). This only leads to unconsciousness and the past madness repeating thoughts and actions which do not serve our higher selves.

The past is comfortable because it is known and familiar; not that it was really "comfortable" or what we wanted.

An imagined or idealized future, while unknown, is a fantasy which usually does not exist where you are right now.

Often we focus on either of these two places because where we are right now according to LS is not what we desire and it is a painful place emotionally in one way or another. We tend to want to avoid the discomfort and pain.

Unfortunately, the only real way to get past discomfort and pain, is to allow yourself to experience it while you move through it. Eventually, you will find you have less of the LS feelings and more of the HS feelings when you allow yourself the grace to get through the negatives.

To live fully be in HS more, which means be fully present to where we are now. We simply slow down, go into our hearts and ask ourselves truly "who am I now and what do I truly want?"

Give up living in your head and instead discover your intuition, trust your gut feelings, and your body. This is the seat of the HS and is a much clearer guide. You can use your intellect as support, to help you build something needed once you know what it is you are called to build.

HS is the ability to see how beautiful, amazing, and perfectly flowing you are, and all is. Through your HS, you will see your vulnerability, mortality, and humanness with gentleness – with LOVE. And this is true security.

When you are living in your HS, you are living now; not yesterday or tomorrow. Now. You can get in touch with this wisdom, love, and joy through following your map and staying on your Walk in Balance journey.

<u>Note</u>: *"In the "Now" is everything. All else is fabricated in our minds: thoughts, feelings, and emotions, which are there to distract us and cause us to repeat the past. Never mind your mind. Instead of thinking, go out in nature, walk, and be quiet; all else will be shown to you. Feel-Be your true self."*

These three distracters are quite amazing, they are like the Zen masters/Sensei's of our life, each day testing us and throwing us to the mat. By overcoming these Distracters, it strengthens us to know our true selves and to know deeply we are one with God. We are never apart. Our challenge is to become so awakened that we are no longer thrown out of balance, but we are in mastery of our own joy, self-love, and peace (HS)!

The solution to distracters is twofold: understanding self-awareness (really be alert to know thyself) and self-management (use self-knowledge/life knowledge to make wise choices). Also known as Emotional intelligence.

We can take a moment now, be brave and identify which of the three is our primary wound. Review the three and determine if you are thrown off by one more often? Ask others who know you. Use all methods available to create a sound assessment (self-awareness).

See all of the ways that we act it out and hurt ourselves and others' each day. Then through the practices on the following pages (self-management), we can choose the activities that guide us beyond the wound and how we want our lives to be!

It is in our hands to make informed choices! It is in our hands to be honest with ourselves and know that each of us has one of these distracters. Will you see this distracter and do something about it or avoid it and let it continue to throw and defeat you?

On the deck….

Mac: Hang on a second. Bill says to see which of these is our primary wound? I can see all three of those happening with me, but not all at the same time. It changes depending upon the situation and the people I'm dealing with.

Sybrian: That can happen. In one situation, you could be seeking approval; in another, control. I think everyone has all three, but usually there is one that tends to be dominant regardless of the circumstances. If you had to pick one, which would it be?

Mac: Hmm….I think seeking approval would be my primary.

Sybrian: What makes you say that?

Mac: Well, in most situations, if I'm trying to take control, it's to make sure things are done so I get approval from someone. And my personal feelings of security are tied to getting the approval of someone, whether it's Betty, my boss, my friends, and such.

Sybrian: It's pretty cool to be able to identify it, isn't it?

Mac: Yep. Now that I'm aware of it, I can see if I am doing something based on what someone else wants just to gain their approval or if it's something I really want. I think that's going to be interesting to watch for and I can see how it might change some of the things I do. Or at least, I'll know "why" I'm doing them.

Sybrian: Awesome! Now, let's go to the next part. I think you'll find this even more interesting.

Control Dramas

In the previous section, I alluded to control dramas. Here is a brief outline of what those are and how we, as human beings use them to gain energy from others.

James Redfield's classic, <u>The Celestine Prophecy,</u> is an excellent read on how to fill yourself up energetically. He offers several ways (9 insights) to connect to natural energy, including meditations on receiving energy from the earth.

He also offers us four dimensions of what he calls "energy dramas" (Lower Self stuff). These are ways people inadvertently 'steal' energy from others if they haven't found/were taught a way to fill themselves directly. These dramas cause a great deal of pain for many people. Dramas create a losing battle for energy and create many of the problems people have in relationships of all types.

<u>The four control dramas are:</u>

"**Poor Me**" This battle steals energy by playing the victim, and subtly getting others to fix them to give them energy.

"**Aloof**" This battle steals energy by acting mysterious and distant, - a ruse to get others to approach them to energize themselves through "look at me, how special I am."

"**Interrogator**" This battle steals energy by constant probing, asking, inquiring about someone's behavior, seeking to control others.

"**Intimidator**" This battle steals energy by bullying and using aggression as a way to take others' power and energy.

I suggest you explore to see if any of these have shown up in your life. Work to fill yourself up with positive energy. Be Authentic with others by being direct when you need to be (asking for what you need, setting boundaries, etc.) while being compassionate with yourself (and others). John Gray's book, <u>What You Can Feel, You Can Heal</u>, also explores dramas and characters people create to avoid their authentic self.

And may I add, as you learn these aspects go easy, for the LS ego mind loves to shame, blame and beat you up for all your stuff. Don't let him. Accept and Create.

Summary Questions-Exercises:

1. Which Distracter gets you?

2. How will you overcome this?

For me, in the name of authenticity and openness, the distracter of 'approval' is my LS wound (addiction). Those with the Approval wound can begin to give to ourselves what we need that is, self-approval, be gentle with ourselves, and be around others who will be too. The 12 step program of Co-Dependence Anonymous was a huge help for me in dealing with this wound, as were various kinds of therapy-healing and coaching. For those in control addiction, learn to stay in union with people, and stop fighting them, allow life to show you how it works for you. For those who are in security addiction, return to trusting life (practice acceptance & creation) to break the spell of judging everyone/thing as wrong.

Back on Deck….

Mac: Whoa!! Okay, that definitely hits a chord!

Sybrian: How so?

Mac: When you put the primary distracter together with the control drama…that's a big eye opener for me!

Sybrian: Tell me!

Mac: Okay, remember that I told you I wasn't going to show Betty the little backyard retreat area until it was done?

Sybrian: Yes…

Mac: There's a reason for it.

Sybrian: I thought you just wanted to surprise her.

Mac: That's what I was telling myself, but that's not true. Not at all. I'm trying to avoid what I think her primary distracter is, protect myself in regards to my primary distracter, and not create control drama! I see that now.

Sybrian: That's a whole lot of LS you've got there. Tell me more.

Mac: I'm going to tell you about another outside project first. This was back when we had made the plans to put the original deck on the back of the house. We planned it and budgeted out the money for it, but we had money left when I went to buy the materials, so I got stuff to build a tree house for the kids because I thought it would be pretty cool.

Sybrian: Did you talk to her about it at all?

Mac: Nope. I ordered the deck materials to be delivered for the weekend, but I took the tree house stuff home in my truck and started on it right away. She came home, saw the tree house and exploded. I didn't have a chance to say a thing.

Sybrian: So, what happened?

Mac: We almost got divorced.

Sybrian: Over a tree house?

Mac: No. Not really. I see now what happened. I wish I knew about all this stuff back then. It would have saved a lot of bad feelings and stress.

Sybrian: Go on...

Mac: Hmm....okay. I'll start with the primary distracters. My primary distracter is the need for approval. I think hers is the need for security. She's always worried about money, but we've never suffered any lack or not been able to do things we want because of money. It's been tight a few times, but we weathered it.

Sybrian: Okay, go on...

Mac: When she was a kid, there was nothing but lack. They often had the power turned off or almost no food in the house because there wasn't enough money.

Sybrian: That could set up a big primary distracter for her, even if that's no longer a problem.

Mac: So the tree house that we didn't discuss set off her primary distracter. She reacted emotionally from her LS without trying to understand first from her HS. Then the control dramas kicked in.

Sybrian: (laughing) Mac, you're fast becoming a pro at this! Keep going.

Mac: So, with the garden retreat, by not talking to Betty about it before I start, I'm actually setting both of us up to fall right back into the same control dramas fueled by our primary distracters. I see that now.

Sybrian: Yep. That's going to create the potential for a whole lot of LS. What are you going to do now that you are aware of these primary distracters and control dramas?

Mac: I'm not really sure. I'm thinking I might need to talk to Betty and show her my idea about the garden retreat before I do anything else.

Sybrian: That's a great idea, but it sounds like you're still feeling some fear and doubt. And you are still operating from your LS with your primary distracter as your base.

Mac: For sure!

Sybrian: How about this? Let's go ahead and finish this chapter since it deals with obstacles, especially fear and doubt. It might help you figure a few more things out. Then we'll stop for the day. Okay?

Mac: Okay, sounds good.

Other Obstacles

Through this Challenge phase, you may discover other obstacles, fears, the LS in many disguises. You may have trauma or PTSD or other deep emotional healing to do, find an appropriate therapist and heal. You may find you have issues with resources such as time, money, and knowledge. The temptation with all issues is to see them as external to you, yet they are internal awaiting your loving attention.

Overall, follow the processes-the Map in the chapters ahead and see what Shifts come from it (meaning it starts with you doing the work, and if you need help reach out to us for some Shift coaching support). Remember Accept and Create. As you Accept: embrace HS, letting go of any need to control how you will obtain the resources you need (or anything for that matter) all is well mindset, and Create: affirm and act on creating what you need with ease and positive energy. You start to see how all your resource needs always "appear" just as you need it.

This is usually because you have released your resistance, your LS demands of what it "should be" and now in HS you trust Great Spirit. You might also begin to see other opportunities and resources you might not have considered previously. They had always been there for you, you just didn't see them.

This may be in the form of a person helping or teaching you how to do something or someone gives you something which you need to take the next step. Or a book or course, the perfect one, presents itself, etc. HS is a power attractor. With HS, you enter flow, synchronicity, and good comes to you.

It's also worth noting that many obstacles are not real; we just perceive them as real. Often, we create obstacles which do not exist at all. We do this because we allow fear, doubt, and worry take over. The LS need for drama feels real and your ego mind will tell you that they are real.

Have you ever experienced this, a time you were so sure someone was doing you wrong, only to find out eventually you were 'making stuff up'? In sum, don't let your LS stop you from living your HS life! In order to get past these fear-based obstacles, you need to face them.

Fears and Doubts

Watch for fears and doubts as they arise each day, await them with courage and compassion; and learn to identify them as what they are. Feel what you need to feel, and then always move forward.

Be Self-Aware and ever alert. Look the fears straight in the eye and say, 'I love you, what do you have to teach me?' LISTEN. Often they say nothing, for they are not real! Or if you hear a true response, say thank you, I hear you and I will do what you need. If it's just LS noise, I now release you to Great Spirit with love, I let you go – I take back my power.' Hence, energetically with love, you embrace them into your heart and work with them - Or slice them out of your life with your samurai sword; Bowing to them for coming to serve you. With HS, you learn how to work with your LS hurts, talking to, listening, loving, learning, releasing and letting go.

Use STOP-Challenge-Choose! A simple Shift formula.
Stop – Pay attention, and as stuff comes up (negative thoughts, feelings, stress) unplug and shift your energy away from habitual lower self-thinking and feeling.
Challenge – Enter the now of HS, Breathe, Relax and Ask what am I thinking that is causing discord? How else can I think, be, in this moment (to bring peace, joy, balance)?
Choose – Choose a higher more powerful way to think and Be (higher self) right now...

One More Thing to Keep in Mind…

Remember not to get mad about all this distraction testing. Stay calm, bow to the Sensei, the teacher (distracter), he is here to strengthen you, to teach you not to give away your power (HS) to these distracters or to anything outside you. See it as an initiation. This is the Hero's Journey. Living your life in all the 'wrong places', till you choose again and come home to HS.

If you are being tested on the hero's journey and you did not know it, you may think you are going insane or the universe is punishing us. Again don't shame yourself or God. The only way out is to pick yourself up and to pass the tests by ascending to your higher self and your higher vibration. Pray often, get help if you need it. It's a wild and wonderful ride. Stay on the journey. Don't let it get you down. God gave you spiritual dynamite to conquer all, use it! Now is the time to ignite the flame within!

Summary Questions:

1. What obstacles are you facing now in moving towards creating your intentions?

    Are they outside, inside, real obstacles or are they roadblocks you have created in your mind?

2. How are/will you moving/move past these obstacles?

3. Test your reasons "why" you want what you want against your obstacles. If you feel your obstacles are insurmountable, you may need to seek stronger reasons "why". Find the deepest, most heartfelt "why" possible.

4. What new things have you been able to discover (resources, opportunities, helpers) by letting go of what you believe for finding solutions to overcome real obstacles?

5. Remember to follow your Map with your daily practice of meditation or prayer, exercise, and journaling.

6. Whenever you find yourself in a LS operating base, remember to STOP-Challenge-Choose.

Back at the house…..

Sybrian: You're awfully quiet. Tell me what you are thinking. I noticed you were jotting down some notes while I was reading. Were you doing the exercises?

Mac: Not yet, but sort of. I mean, It's all really interesting, and I'm sort of understanding it, but I'm not really sure how I can make it work for me. It seems sort of complicated.

Sybrian: Okay, what do you want to know?

Mac: How does it all fit together to create the outcome you want?

Sybrian: You mean, "How are you going to create the garden retreat the way you want it to be without upsetting Betty about how much money it will cost?" Is that right?

Mac: Yes.

Sybrian: Okay. Let's start here. You've pretty much determined what your primary distracter is and which one is hers. Both are LS and fear based; the fear creates your doubt in approaching her about the project at all. Right?

Mac: Right, because of how much it will cost and I don't want another tree house control drama with all the bad feelings that go with it.

Sybrian: Do you remember what Bill said about "being present" with the current situation rather than being in the past or the future?

Mac: Yes.

Sybrian: The tree house is in the past; the garden is in the future.

What is your "now" which you have to work through? It's the painful part you have to work through in order to create a higher vibrational frequency.

Mac: My "now" is... I am going to have to talk to Betty and show her what I want to do in the garden. I have to face my own doubts and fears in a way that honors and respects hers.

Sybrian: WOW! Exactly! That is operating from your HS!

Mac: But I don't know how to do it!

Sybrian: (sighs) We were almost there. LS is a low vibrational energy. Doubt is LS. Control is LS. Which means, even looking for "How" is a need for control.

Mac: So, I need to let go of the "how"?

Sybrian: Yes.

Mac: I don't understand. I can't do the project without working on how to talk to Betty and how to do the work itself without costing a lot of money!

Sybrian: First, let go of the need for acceptance, approval, and security. Next, "park" your control dramas. Then, while you are meditating and praying, see and feel the garden retreat as finished. See and feel you and Betty sitting out there, having a good time, laughing and enjoying it together. Feel your love for her and put that into the garden space as well.

Mac: I don't understand how that will help me create the garden and not upset Betty.

Sybrian: You said you were going to "think on it" anyway, so would it hurt to try this?

Mac: I guess not.

Sybrian: Didn't you say you already feel a lot better and things are going more smoothly for you overall since you started with Walk in Balance with me?

Mac: Yes, but I really don't see how this is going to work. That fish pond is going to be expensive and Betty isn't going to like that.

Sybrian: That's your LS talking. Doubt, fear...they are both right there.

Mac: I know! But I can't see how...ugh. I just did it again!

Sybrian: (laughing) No worries. It takes time to move out of your LS. Have a little faith. Give it a chance to work.

Mac: Okay. What about that "Law of Attraction" stuff? Can I get a free fountain with it?

Sybrian: Maybe. But don't limit the LoA by expecting a "free fountain" to appear. Leave the possibilities open.

Mac: This. Is. Crazy. I should just work some overtime for the money.

Sybrian: No. That is in direct conflict with your intentions and priorities.

Mac: You said this was simple.

Sybrian: It is simple; just not always easy. How about this: Just give it a chance. Meditate, play, work on keeping your vibrational energy high. Keep working on the project, but don't spend any money on it yet. Wait for the answers or resources to reveal themselves to you. They will come to you.

Mac: Okay. I'm going to keep meditating, praying, following my map, journaling...and do the exercises. I'm going to visualize Betty sitting with me by the fish pond and enjoying it.

Sybrian: Now, what about talking to Betty about the project and showing her the garden retreat area?

Mac: I'm going to have to work up to that. I'm going to need to talk to her without triggering her primary distracter. That's a "how" I don't have.

Sybrian: Okay, but what if you do?

Mac: Right now, I don't know that either.

Sybrian: Actually, I think you do know. Make that part of your meditation. Maybe it will help you find your answers.

Mac: Okay. I'll do it. I don't know how it's going to help, but...

Sybrian: There you go with "how" again! Let it go!

Mac: Right. Okay. Let go of all the "how" questions and the LoA is just going to bring me the answers. Pfft. Right.

Sybrian: (laughing) Give up your need to control. Let it happen. Let's meet at the end of the week. Call me if you get stuck on something or need to talk before then.

Mac: Will do!

Phone Call...
Mac: You are not going to believe this!

Sybrian: Well, hello, Mac! Try me. I might.

Mac: Okay, remember the promotion I'd been trying to get?

Sybrian: Yes.

Mac: I got it!

Sybrian: Congrats!

Mac: Believe it or not, never taking time off and working all those extra hours was what was keeping me from getting promoted! My boss said that they like their key people to have "more balanced lives." Once I started taking a couple of personal days to work in my garden, they decided I had figured it out.

Sybrian: "Walk In Balance"!

Mac: Yep! And I talked to Betty.

Sybrian: How did that go?

Mac: Since I had the promotion, I decided to work up the plans and the costs for the garden. When I showed it to her, she actually liked it. She was a little worried about the cost and wanted me to skip the waterfall, so I agreed to go with the cheaper fountain instead.

Sybrian: Cool!

Mac: But then, something else happened and now, the waterfall is going to be built instead.

Sybrian: What happened?
Mac: Totally unbelievable. Just after Betty and I finished talking about the garden and I agreed to the fountain, our next door neighbor rang the doorbell.

Sybrian: And???

Mac: His wife saw the flower boxes and loved them. He wanted to know if I would build some for his wife AND make a few as gifts for a couple of his landscaping customers. What he offered to pay for them was enough to make up the difference between the fountain and the waterfall!

Sybrian: That's Awesome!!

Mac: So, you were right about letting go, keeping my vibrational energy high, relaxing, and trying to find ways to enjoy my life instead of working all the time! This LoA stuff...Walk In Balance...IT WORKS! I feel great!

Sybrian: Great! But, you know...there's more...

Mac: Now you sound like those TV ads! There's more?

Sybrian: Well, yes. We haven't gotten to the end of the book yet.

Mac: Oh, right. Okay, what's next? I can't wait to see where this goes from here!

Sybrian: The next part is Healing.

Mac: Healing? Didn't we already talk about overcoming energy dramas and obstacles?

Sybrian: Yes, sort of. But in order to truly Walk in Balance, you have to go deeper into your Core Processes.

Mac: Core Processes? What are those?

Sybrian: Core Processes are what we do each day to bring ourselves more and more into living from our Higher Self.

Mac: Isn't that what I am already doing with meditation and journaling?

Sybrian: That's part of it, but there's more. Don't worry. It's fun and easy. The best part is, you will find yourself living a more joyful life, filled with what you love doing and being. Does that sound good to you?

Mac: With as good as I am feeling and as well as everything is going, if I can have more of that, of course it sounds good to me!

Sybrian: Great! You are already on your way! So, read the next chapter and I'll meet you for lunch in a few days.

The Peace of the Wild Things

When despair for the world grows in me and I wake in the middle of the night at the least sound in fear of what my life and my children's lives may be, I go lie down where the wood drake rests in his beauty on the water, and the great Heron feeds.

I come into the peace of wild things who do not tax their lives with forethought of grief. I come into the presence of still water. And I feel above me the day-blind stars waiting for their light. For a time I rest in the grace of the world, and I am free.

- *Wendell Berry*

Chapter 5: Healing and the Core Process

We are what we accept and create each day. Over the years, these days add up to make a life. We are either masters or dabblers of this journey of HS. Life is far too short to dabble, and to be trapped and hurt in the trance of LS. The joy of life is in the moment, in each day, daring to be our true self.

Most of us are out of balance in that we work 18 hours a day, sleep seven and have -1 hour for life. We have no time for Self. We need to make some changes here! How about reduce work hours (to some manageable level), sleep seven hours, and have 9 or so hours for loving ourselves, our family and living life. Otherwise, where has our life gone?

Isn't it wonderful to know that there is an incredible universe conspiring for your greatness? Affirm: 'I am a Gift to this World... I deserve to be happy, alive, joyful and abundant. All I need comes to me with grace and ease as I live in me. The universe is a miracle and so am I."

We have now arrived at Stage 3 of the Medicine Wheel which is Healing.
Stage 1 is Vision: what do you want?
Stage 2 is Challenge-Chaos: how do I overcome the challenge of the three distracters?

Stage 3 is Healing: Using Unity, Energy, and Impeccability (the Core Process) to more fully live your true HS life.
In this stage of Healing, we are going to go deeper into our daily lives, to add things which bring us more joy, Love and HS. You will be connecting with your spirituality, creating more positive energy, and discovering new understanding.

Here are some suggestions for living the plan, more in your HS, happy throughout the day, and keeping your vibration high! Keep it simple. Find a way to take 20 minutes each morning and evening for meditation and prayer. Then, work your way up to an hour or whatever feels right for you. Practice this each day. In time, you will feel so good.

I know what some of you are thinking. You are thinking your schedule and your life are overfull and there is absolutely no way you are going to "find" the extra 15 to 30 minutes, twice a day, to meditate.

"You should sit in meditation for 20 minutes each day... Unless you are too busy; Then you should sit for an hour."
~Zen Proverb

Take care of yourself first (This is the foundation of this book). Then support others (start with you then share like the oxygen mask in an airplane!). Meditate and use the Core Processes every day. Your life will change, and as you change, your priorities will change. You will become an example of the new man, the new woman – Walking in Balance.

Daily Core Practices: Unity, Energy, and Impeccability
Some examples for you to choose from...

I. Unity: *Staying connected to HS (Love)*
Meditation: *20 minutes each morning and night*
Sit quietly each morning for twenty minutes and again before bed. Count your breaths and say the following:
The peace of God is flowing through me now (The Love of God, The Joy God or similar, whatever feels comfortable to you); after ten minutes release words and just concentrate your breathing. Release, be, reject nothing... simply allow what comes. See thoughts and worry as 'thinking' and let it go – stay in the peace of now.

When you first start this practice, see how the mind tries to 'run' us, especially when we try to unplug from it. Meditation is the foundational practice of several of the world's religions because it is the best way to enter HS.

Use the following tips to help your meditation fun:

- Sit quietly, sacred place, straight back, cross legs (If you cannot sit like this, find a comfortable position in which to sit).

- Relax your muscles....close your eyes if you wish.

- Be aware of your breath as it flows in and out through nostrils.

- Another wonderful meditation mantra:
  On the inhale say, "Breathing in... calm my mind and body." On the exhale say, "Breathing out... I release and I trust."

- Go slow, calm, watch...let go of any thoughts which return to words, breathe...relax...

- When you're done take some minutes to Pray, say the Rosary, do mantras (repeating sacred words)...connect with Spirit in the way which works best for you and fits in with your beliefs.

- In the language of your own heart ask for assistance on your earth walk and for all on the planet with us.

- Pray for protection, surround yourself with white light, and smudge with sage frequently. Keep an altar nearby with meaningful objects, pictures, and candles. Embrace sacredness.

- Affirm - Just for today: I will be Grateful, Loving. I will do my work honestly. I will be Kind to every living thing and all people! I will walk in beauty and light. Add others as you like.

Presencing (meaning being Present always) When not 'in meditation', use this practice to stay in the HS, gain guidance, and be present any time you need it.

1. Pay attention to your inner state and **Unplug** from any of your Lower self and all the anger, worry, and upset of your mind's whining of things we cannot control or of what someone else is doing. Just unplug, drop it, cut it, and let it go. If you are really triggered, remember to practice riding the wave. Do nothing but be present: Breathe, Relax, Feel, Watch, and Allow. This can be intense when a wound, past trauma or distractor is activated.

2. **Enter** your Higher self (Presence), the older, wiser, and calm soul within us. Take a few minutes to Breathe deeply, Pray, Become quiet and calm down. Center yourself. Everything is happening for a reason. Be brave and enter into trust. If you are able, go outside and connect with nature to help.

3. **Inquire** with your higher self for guidance as needed. What is needed now? What is the highest path here? Note all options and choose the best with what you CAN do. All you can do is all you can do, and all you can do, is enough! Act on what you are capable of and let the rest go.

A close cousin to STOP-Challenge-Choose! (Chapter 4)

II. Energy: *Staying connected to HS, with Vibrancy, Aliveness*

Move, Breathe, Eat right

Daily Energizing practices
(for more, see the WIB Life Energy E-Book practice guide)

Move: Move your body to raise your energy. Walk, yoga, swim, team sports...whatever works for you. You choose. Do some type of physical activity for 30 minutes day. Sweat a little. It is good for you! There is no need to overdo it. Be gentle and consistent. Stretch more and more as you can. Please see your doctor before beginning any exercise program. Take it easy...

Deep Breaths: (2 x a day) in car or in transit take (10) - (3) parts yogic breaths to energize body and release toxins: Inhale slowly and fully to a count of (7), Hold to count of (7), Exhale slowly to count of (7). Do (10) of these (3) part full breaths and you will feel like a million bucks!

Nutrition: Eat plenty of color (green, yellow, red and blue etc.) foods; If you can, choose organic foods (pesticide, antibiotic, and hormone free) over non-organic. Drink plenty of clean water and limit caffeine and alcohol. Also limit your intake of meat and processed foods. Your diet should be at least 50% water content, meaning fruits and veggies. Reduce non-water content foods such as breads; and limit meats to less than 10 oz. per day. Eat nothing that is white. Get help from a competent professional nutritionist to test you for the right diet. Find a balance between healthy fats, carbs, and proteins. Important!!!! No more sodas; drink water!

Sweeteners (when you need): Agave Nectar, Organic Maple Syrup, Natural Fructose, and Splenda.

Snacks: Organic Energy Bars, (A good source: **www.activegreens.com**) Raw Almonds, Dates, Blue Berries, Asia or Gobi Berry, Blue Corn Chips with Organic Guacamole! Yum... and good for you!

Eating Right: Most importantly is HOW you eat. Slow down, eat without distractions (taking your time to fully present with the food) and pray. Speaking Wind taught me this prayer: *"Thank you for coming to me my friend and surrendering your life that I may continue mine."* Eating is a sacrament. Enter it consciously. And chew; masticate each bite 30 times before swallowing or you will be doing violence on your digestive track. Slow down and enjoy!

Sleep: Get proper rest. If you don't get enough sleep at night, for whatever reason, try to take naps when you can. Sleep is important to your overall well-being.

Cleanse periodically: First timers, find a guide to support you through this detoxification process.

Augment these with Essential Oils, Herbs, Smudging, and Prayer

Diet and Nutrition: Bill's Personal Notes

These are things I have used and have been successful for me. There are many great resources here for great products which have contributed to my own Path and Core Practices.

Cleansing the Body

Cleanse periodically. It is preferred that you cleanse with medical supervision. I have used Dr. Shulze's Isagenix. Isagenix is a 30 day cleanse which Dr. Shulze recommends twice per year to detoxify your body and lose weight naturally. (Dr. Schultze: https://www.herbdoc.com)
You can also try this 'Ultimate', cleanse for a week: Water, Cayenne Pepper, lots of squeezed lemons and a bit of Maple syrup... cleans you out! Like an oil change and tune up for your body! Experiment and add golden-seal or other herbs to help flush the liver, kidneys, and colon. First timers, find a guide to support you through this detoxification process.

See your doctor, Naturopath, Holistic healing profession or Nutritionist for guidance on products, procedure, and any health concerns before starting any cleanse.

I also recommend Young Living Essential Oils: (for vitality) anoint yourself on head and neck and other places as needed. You can get a starter kit and experiment. Deeply cleansing, relaxing, energizing... amazing!
www.youngliving.com

My best nutritional day:

7:30 am: After waking, *Super Green Shake and Green tea or sometimes wheat-grass, try it. It is one of the most nutritional products on earth!

9:45 am: 2 scrambled eggs with organic spinach (sometimes Organic Oatmeal with protein powder, dash of maple syrup and banana)

12:30 pm: Lunch: Live Organic Salad (with nuts, sprouts, assorted veggies) with 4 oz Wild Salmon, Iced Tea

7:00 pm: Dinner: Bowl of fresh Soup, 1 slice of Ezekiel Bread, Organic Brown Rice w/Organic Broccoli and Carrots (sometimes Tomatoes, Yellow Squash). Add 3 oz. of fish or protein source as needed. Hot tea. On occasion, enjoy a glass of Red Wine or Dark Chocolate for desert.

***Super Green Shake:** 1 large table spoon of Greens Plus – super food powder, in water with 1 dropper Bach Rescue Remedy, great for reducing overall stress , 1 dropper Supreme Echinacea-Golden Seal , for immune strength, from www.GaiaHerbs.com 1 dropper Quantum Male Energy Formula (Female for ladies,) this is for overall Strength, ... mix and drink. Sometimes add 1000mg Vitamin C (1 packet Emerge-C). Supplement with other needed essential vitamins/herbs for added boost! All supplements listed above are in most Natural Health food stores.*

When I am not feeling well: I drink Green shake with 3000 mg Vitamin C (powder) 3 x per day, take fluids & rest, minimize or eliminate other food for a while. It will knock out most ailments. Add garlic for extra kick.

Also, purchase the Natural Herb book (see resources at back of book) and become familiar with many amazing natural remedies that medicine people have been using for centuries. This will help with most physical challenges such as headaches, cramps, fever, colds, etc... Some are put in teas, or chewed, or come in liquid form to add to drinks. See web sites for www.GaiaHerbs.com or Quantum Herbs.

See a competent Naturopath/Homeopath, Chinese doctor, Medicine person, Reiki Master, Acupuncture, Shamanic Practices, Healing Body Work, Cranial Sacral,

Chiropractic, or professional Therapist to guide you. Keep list of practitioners in your area.

Please go to a Western medical doctor or other trusted Heath professional if symptoms of low energy, and fatigue etc. persist!

Recommended Products:

Greens Plus: Green-Berry drink (for AM drink) from *www.greensplus.com*

Oasis Meta Greens and **Meta Berry** (alternative to above): *www.oasislifescieces.com*

Green Vibrance: http://www.vibranthealth.us/

Amazon Herb Company: Digestive Enzymes for lunch & dinner to help assimilate food ... vital after age of 45. www.amazonherb.net

Peaceful Planet Energy Shake: (www.Neutriceutical.com). *For Protein Boost. And many others: Warrior Blend, Hemp.*

Bach Rescue Remedy, Flower Essences for Health & Energy (Whole foods)

Snacks: Organic Energy Bars: www.activegreens.com

Always seek the advice of a health professional when making changes to your diet or activity level (exercise). Make sure that any natural or herbal supplements do not conflict with any prescription medications you may already be taking.

Other Energy:

Mind / Words: Speak cleanly and only what is true. Count your Blessings! Avoid gossip, worry, and negativity. Be positive.

Action / Initiative: Take Initiative when needed; otherwise wait for the right moment. Be Patient. Balance Non-doing and doing.

Bonding with others: Connect. **Love someone today.**

Reverence for all: humans, animals, nature, earth.

Body / Play: Use your body and play instead of living in mind chatter / thought. The magic is in letting go and letting it come; over thinking only gets in the way. Treat your body with ultimate respect. Eat right, move, and breathe! Ask your body what is true and follow the guidance of your heart. Have some fun!

Clearing: Smudging (Blessing the body and aura with the smoke of sage blends.). Bathe yourself in white Light.

III. Impeccability: *Stay connected to HS (Strength of Focus)*

"Where the Attention goes… the Energy flows."

- **Read** your Map/Intentions to stay on track (3 minutes each morning)
- **Ask** your Intentions "what do you need from me today?" Act on what you need.
- **Read and Integrate** the Seven Principles of Life at lunchtime each day for (3) minutes. (next page)
- **Read good books to feed your Spirit** each evening for at least 20 minutes.

- **Cleanse** yourself and release the day before Bed. Sage, meditation, prayer. Journal any thoughts, ideas.

Speaking Wind's, *Seven Principles of Life*:
(From: The Way of the Corporate Shaman)

1. Find the part of you that lives in all things. What is your path? Find it, Live it!
2. Let self-doubt and self-pity fall away. Live in HS!
3. Place yourself first, before all things and all others. If you don't take care of you, who will?
4. Look at the negative emotions for what they have to teach you. Everything is a teacher! Listen!
5. Allow all things to "be". Relax...It's all working out!
6. Life is to understand and to learn...not to control. Life is an adventure in discovery, so enjoy it! None of us have it figured out!
7. The child grows; the adult only grows old. Be youthful, playful, and have fun!

Use As Needed (when emotional stuff is up ..)

Conscious Reframing – Self Forgiveness
(Awareness, Forgiveness, Rebirth)

Whenever you recognize something happening in your world that you do not want (i.e., the LS emotional grip), Enter **Awareness** (witness). Accept that you created it, (or at least that it is a part of you...your LS). Own it. Be responsible for your creation. See the pattern as it comes up and acknowledge it, even laugh at it. No one is doing it to you. Out of compassion, your true self is bringing you the pattern repeatedly, until you truly understand it. Be loving and patient with self.

Next, **Forgive** yourself for that creation. Keep releasing any judgments about yourself. Stop feeding it (the LS) by unplugging the power cord - do not give it juice. Instead, let go. Look deeply at and into the core of the emotion, go right to its center, and just be <u>Present</u> to it. It simply wants your attention, to talk to you. You can do this without being taken over by it. This will diffuse the energy. A gift will be given to you.

Once you start to feel calm and empowered, **Rebirth** yourself. Choose your thoughts, feelings, and actions according to your true desires. To be free, to feel good, etc. Ask yourself, "What do I really want in this moment?" and go with that. You can choose that, try it on for size, and see how it fits you. You are in control of your mind and body. You have the power! God is in you.

Repeat these steps as many times as you need in order to move yourself out of LS. If you feel stuck or you are in pain, find a local healer, counselor or helper who can support you in person.

Use some version of this to forgive others if they have hurt you. Example: "I love you, I release you to the Holy Spirit; I take back our power!"

Affirmations

Affirmations can be used daily, several times a day. Many people use them as part of their morning, noon, and/or night core processes. There are different ways to use affirmations. You can say them as part of or after your meditation. You can say them in the mirror. You can sing them in the car on the way to work. Affirmations are powerful supporting statements of who you are and what you want. Say them with energy and feeling. Love the words. Energize them. Affirmations help you realign your thought patterns to the positive and help you break any old, negative thought patterns which you may be stuck in, out of habit.

Mike Dooley (tut.com) says, "Thoughts are things, so think the good ones!" Your self-talk, including your thoughts, are part of your conversation with God and the universe. It is part of your energy. It influences what you create in your life and draw to you.

Here are some ideas for affirmations for you to use. Or, create your own! You can speak, sing, and dance your affirmations wildly. Give them energy! Bring them to life!

This is a really fun example of affirmations on YouTube: https://www.youtube.com/watch?v=qR3rKOkZFkg (a video of a little girl named Jessica. Her affirmations are lively, fun, and full of positive energy.)

Here are some sample affirmations you can use:

I am a gift to the world; I deserve to be happy, healthy, whole, and abundant.
I am entitled to feel good
I am entitled to miracles - I am a Miracle
I am at the right place at the right time!
I am safe to be powerful
I am on purpose
I can have now what I intend
All is well, I feel great... no matter what
And it's ok to feel and be real
I am clearing the past and stepping into my future
I reclaim my power
Love and Trust is the way I walk
I know at times my mind can't understand, I relax, I send my mind peace.
I ask the God source to bring me peace
I choose to know I am safe
I breathe deeply into myself, I can relax
I nurture myself with calm, peace, love, well-being.

Joy and Peace to me
It's ok to trust, all is well!
The more I rest and nurture myself...
The more I draw to myself the perfect resources, people, and gifts.
Worry shuts me off, I choose otherwise.
God source give me a direct experience of presence; I relax learn, listen, be... with ease.
I choose now the grounding of myself in safety... all is well.
And from this safety I soar to new heights of joy
I am Co-Creator of my world... I choose beauty
My gifts, talents are used now in stimulating, fun, rewarding work, in balance.
I am healthy
I request what I want....and ask the universe to provide... I want_____ _____
_____

I am calm, I speak what I want, the universe provides clear signs to guide me, I am grateful that all my needs are provided for. This or something way better arrives into my life.
I feel good, I feel trust, I can have fun on earth.
I rest and do what I want... and only act from inspired action, not force
I know what to do... Stop, breathe, consolidate... and affirm all is well.
I know exactly what to do to create...
All my needs are met easily... I am free... financially, personally... free.
I am full of joy, peace... I am on Purpose.
I place my order, I know It is on its way now
I joyfully receive
I dial up my inner GPS (intuition) and follow her guidance on where to go, what to do, what to say and to whom...

I allow my core self (HS) to lead

I am fine, I am supported, miracles are flowing as my ever day reality

I am Beautiful, I am Amazing

I am valuable, I am worthy

I am love and light

I allow in what is possible

I am supported in trying anew, experimenting, taking risks, dancing, stepping into the unknown..

The universe always provides me with a gentle cushion... I am safe and secure

I am open to what is next...wow

My life is filled with love and joy. I love my life...it is amazing

I allow amazing windfalls to come to me constantly!

Have a beautiful loving life, with balance of work and play.

I create my world...my world is beautiful and joyful

Plenty of time for me, stimulating work when I want it... and financial independence!

It is done... I am so Grateful for all I have, all I give, and all I receive.

The daily practices are key recommended fundamentals, a core process (Pull from these in creating part your final draft of your Life Map, chapter 6). Start here and never let a day pass without enjoying the gift you are giving yourself! God gave you spiritual dynamite to conquer all, use it! Now is the time to ignite the flame within!

More...

Weekly Core Practices

While the daily practices are the foundation, a couple times per week you can augment with coaching and/or gatherings, etc. Which of these could you do each week to live fully, to support your path? If these don't "feel" right to you, what can you choose for yourself to help you better live from your HS? To live in Joy?

1. Participate in weekly Inspirational meetings for community, support, understanding the way, and inspiration! Find a tribe (group of like-minded people) and get together on a topic of interest! Go to weekly Prosperity groups, Masterminds, CPDA Groups, Meet Ups, Religious study groups, churches, etc.

2. Engage in Nature / earth medicine pursuits: Nature is a teacher. It is so wonderful to walk in the woods, on the beach, or even sit by a river. Being in nature clears our mind and renews us. All of life is healing. Water, earth, fire, air, all beings/creatures are healing elements. These parts of the circle sustain us; Respect and pay attention to what they can teach us and how they can energize us. Go outside in nature to watch, look, and listen. Animals... watch them in silence. What do they tell you? Water and fire...observe them, let them teach you. Learn about plant medicines, the power of all nature and her energy healing.

Sun Bear's books (and many other top Native American medicine people's books) offer many ancient 'recipes' for using healing herbs and plants to help us return to balance. Air... breathe her in and be grateful for breath! Play with the rock people of the earth and feel their power to heal. Drink water; sit in a hot steam/spring or cool river...these are very healing. Sit in the sun for a few minutes and absorb needed nutrients. Have fun letting life and nature teach you something new!

3. See a coach/counselor to work on Shifting your stuff:

Trans-personal/ depth Psychotherapy (Jungian)
Shift 'Walk in Balance' Coaching with Bill or Sybrian
Neuro Linguistic Programming
Emotional Freedom Technique and Sedona Method
Body Centered/Phoenix Rising Yoga Therapy
Behavior Based Life Path Coaching
Shamanism Ceremony, Energy work
Past Life Therapy

Working with a Coach will boost your well-being and success to be the best you can be! It is the best investment you will ever make!

4. Use as many Weekly Personal 'wholesome' Happiness rituals as you can. Share these experiences and rituals with those you love! Here are a few ideas, in self-care and love:

Luscious massage and/or energy work.
Hot, bubbly, essential oil and salt bath.
Swim in a lake, ocean, or stream.
Hike a mountain, ride a horse.
Play with animals, kids, hug a tree or loved one.
Dance wild!!! Make Love!
Play sports, sail, roller blade, golf, tennis, canoe, ski, and bike.
Or my favorite: the stressful sport of hammock resting and sipping iced tea... Ah-h-h-h!
See a good movie or a play.
Listen to great music.
Read Poetry. Write Poetry.

Make a sumptuous meal and enjoy with friends.
Have a glass of nice red wine... why not? (Use discretion whenever drinking.)
Plant a garden and play in it each day.
Indulge in Maple Mud Chocolate Peanut Butter... and eat it with a spoon right from the jar! Yum!
Attend classes for yoga, martial arts, dance, acting, art, etc.
Did anyone say Beach? Go surfing... skinny dip, or just sand bathe.
Go to a new town and explore. Visit a museum.
Relax!
Help someone less fortunate; give a smile or a helping hand.
Go Sailing!
Play with your pets.
Foster kittens waiting for adoption.
Rake a big pile of leaves and jump in!
Build a snowman... dance in the rain.
The key is to do as many of your Happiness Rituals as you can each week! Customize to you and enjoy!

(There is a list of resources and books in the back of this book. Check them out and enjoy!)

Monthly Core Practices

What we can do each month to live fully by sharing with others what we have learned.

You can be a leader or help lead in your community a monthly meeting or gathering around the new and full moon with self and others celebrating life, releasing and enjoying tribe!

Key Ceremony/Rituals to share with others at local monthly gatherings:

Sharing Circles (Soul Circle, Master Mind Group)
Journeying
Meditation/Yoga or similar
Conscious listening (use of talking sticks)
Drum/Dance/Music Circle / Chanting/Singing
Group Dinner
Group Hike
Prayer Circle
Satsang wisdom circle
New moon/Full moon gatherings

Earth Blessings: Make medicine gifts and give them to earth/others. You can make medicine bundles, sage-tobacco; sacred giveaways, or anything else your heart feels works for you and your tribe.

Burning the Past Ritual:
Write down all your upsets for the month and then toss the paper into a bonfire to burn them away. Feel the release... feel the freedom... how wonderful. Then affirm and write down what you intend for the next month to replace the old with something new. Sing it, scream it, and dance it. Let it become you!

Quarterly Core Practices

There are many opportunities to expand upon your daily, weekly, and monthly Core Practices.
These will be special times or events which only happen once or a few times per year, such as the Solstice, the Equinox, Blue Moons, and special holidays or dates with personal meaning. The greatest gift we can give to the

earth mother, ourselves, and each other is to gather and bless each other and our planet.

Many of these events are important times of change; others are significant times of reflection and meditation to gain new understanding.

You can attend retreats in nature or at a Holistic Center for rest, renewal, and re-inspiration to bring your vision all together. Some people find balance in religious retreats or camping trips. Other people discover their perfect retreat at the beach or in the mountains. Regardless of your choice, this is a time to give, receive, and bless one another in the world around each Solstice/Equinox.

<u>You may feel called to attend</u>: *with those certified to lead ..*
Pipe Ceremony (Cha'nupa')
Sweat Lodge (Inipi)
Soul Retrieval/Extraction work
Five-day fasting wilderness Vision Quest
Participate in Sun Dance (advanced, by invitation from Lakota nation)

Share the "World 11" adherences
All the world religions-people seem to agree on these:
1. Love all, even what you cannot love.
2. Nonviolence, Non-stealing, Non Possession.
3. Generosity and Kindness.
4. Compassion to those hurting.
5. Balance in all things; Moderation in work, sex, food, etc. Simplicity!
6. Respect all beings, all creatures and Mother Earth.
7. Honesty – Speak only what you know to be true.
8. Walk Gently … and in reverence… leave no trail.
9. Be brave, stand up for what you know is right.
10. Leave each day better than when we started.
11. Trust in God… all is working out for the best

Summary –

There is a lot offered to you in this chapter. Take a moment and pray, and ask HS which to choose (and integrate into your life plan). Keep it simple. A few activities completed joyfully daily are a lot better than many never done.

Start with:

- Meditate and pray each morning.
- Read your Life Map and follow it, affirm it.
- Exercise/Movement (walk, bike, swim, yoga) minimum ___ minutes per day. Smile.
- Journal on your successes and key learnings, then meditate before bed.
- Stay soul connected in weekly spiritual groups. (ongoing)

Another Phone Call....

Mac: Hey there, Sybrian!

Sybrian: Hi, Mac! What's up?

Mac: This section about Healing...

Sybrian: What about it?

Mac: There's a lot in here that really isn't going to work for me.

Sybrian: Like what?

Mac: Vegetarian? Organic? Didn't I see you wolfing down a huge burger at lunch the other day? What's up with that?

Sybrian: Oh...yes. That was a tad off track. The wolfing it down part, I mean. Vegetarian doesn't really work for me, so I don't do that.

Mac: But then you aren't following the Walk in Balance program!

Sybrian: Yes; yes I am.

Mac: How?

Sybrian: Okay, back up a bit. Do you remember way, way back in the beginning of the book where Bill says that if something doesn't fit for you, then it doesn't fit? Like an exercise plan that includes jogging, but you have a bad knee, so it doesn't work for you, so choose something else?

Mac: I remember something like that.

Sybrian: Well, not eating meat does not work for me! Wolfing my food down, well...that's another story. Since we eat lunch together fairly often, you won't have any trouble with this one. You know how you are always saying that I am the "slowest eater on earth"?

Mac: Yeah...

Sybrian: That's because I try to eat slowly, savoring the food, and giving thanks for each bite I put into my mouth. When I ate that burger too fast, it caused me to have some serious indigestion later in the day. I would have been better to have eaten less more slowly.

Mac: Okay, so what you are saying is...do as many of the Core Processes as I am comfortable with.

Sybrian: Yes.

Mac: I'm not into "new moon" and "full moon" ceremonies. Nope. Not at all. That sounds plain demonic to me.

Sybrian: (sighing) Okay, Mac. But before you completely reject them, we should probably have a chat about them sometime. You can say whatever prayers you want when you do the ceremonies, remembering "what fits for you". The ceremonies are about healing. Forgiving, letting go, and sharing that time with others.

Mac: I don't know.

Sybrian: How about this? If you decide you want to try one of the new moon or full moon ceremonies, let me know. We can plan it and you can host it in your garden retreat, if it feels right to you. If not, no worries.

Mac: I'll think about it.

Sybrian: Bottom line is this: Use only the Core Practices which feel right to you and for you. They are about strengthening your HS, not your LS which is what is happening now.

Mac: I'm strengthening my LS?

Sybrian: Yes. Doubt and fear about some of the Core Practices feeds your LS. And you don't even have to use those! Move on to the ones that feel good to you and just use them.

Mac: Okay. I get it.

Sybrian: Great! Do you feel ready to start the next section?

Mac: Yep. As long as I don't have to dance around a bonfire under a full moon in my skivvies.

Sybrian: Mac! Really, now!

Mac: Just kidding. I might like it.

Sybrian: Ugh! Well, at least you're not so grumpy anymore! I can't remember the last time you said anything close to a joke.

Mac: Want to meet for an organic burger on Friday?

Sybrian: Sure! As long as I can take my time and I don't have to listen to stories of you running around in your underwear!

Mac: No worries there. And I'm thinking I should slow down my eating now too.

Sybrian: Good idea! See you then!

How can I Energize and Feel Great Today?

Chapter 6: Walking in Balance

Congratulations!
You have made it to the final phase, stage 4.

Stage 1 is Vision: What do you want?
Stage 2 is Challenge-Chaos: How do I overcome the challenge of the three distracters?
Stage 3 is Healing: Using Unity, Energy, and Impeccability, the core process to more fully live your true HS life.

Stage 4 is Maturity: Mastering the daily path in a sustainable way.

To enter Stage 4: Maturity to our highest expression is an ongoing never-ending fun adventure. We need to exercise the plan (our plan) for one year successfully to earn our first merit badge, then five years for the Eagle Scout, and then a life to enter maturity and be a master. This kind of rigor and discipline (devotion) can be tough... who has the time? I am too busy doing other things!

What I do like, is that it is a relatively easy plan, simple and offers maximum flexibility. There is no 'thou shall' or "thou must" kind of stuff coming from anyone. This is a personal core decision. Ultimate, what happens is that when you begin with the daily practices (slowly), then add the weekly practices (one or two to start with) you build new Walk in Balance habits. Loving commitments to you.

When you do something every day, it becomes easy and a part of your life. It's not about "having enough time". It's about choosing what you want. You get to choose, you know? You choose the way you want to live. So, what is the way you want to live?

Practicing the core processes is sustainable when it serves you and serves the world repeatedly, and when it comes from love. Over time, which of the core processes you use may vary, because as you use them, you change, so they will also change.

For example, the affirmations you use as you begin this process will most likely not be identical to the ones you will be using a year from now. If you choose an exercise plan, it will change as your body changes. Your intentions (some of them) will change as well. This is because as you change, life changes.

So, live fully, honor all, and leave no harm. Even better, live fully and inspire the world to be better because you have lived your best life. And it all starts with taking care of you first!

Based on everything we have discussed, what you have learned, it's time to go back to your notes and previous work on your priorities on how you choose to spend your time (next page). This is an exercise you will re-visit many times over as you grow.

Your Keys Focuses to live your Priorities are?
Complete your Life Plan (Map) Now pg. 108

Great job! Now you have a clear Walk in Balance focus. Go forth. Commit, have fun. I challenge anyone to make the change, to live the core 'self-care' process for one year, and you will see a very transformed person, one that has deeply touched many others, just by being you.

For the Ultimate Challenge, go for two years. This will truly create amazing changes in your life. Take the two-year challenge and see!

All it takes is self-love and dedication to you, by you. Maybe this is the toughest choice of all: to finally put yourself, your true self-first and save the inner world. Have no fear; you are a total giver. Take care of you and watch all the good that your heart can do. You will discover you can do more for others when you have put yourself and your well-being first. Walk in Balance!

Where will 'my time' go, Now?

Create categories and designate hours You CHOOSE Now ...
(in wheel below...)

Work	Self Time	Exercise
Family	Commuting	Sleeping
Service	Adventure	Learning
Spiritual	Socializing	Other

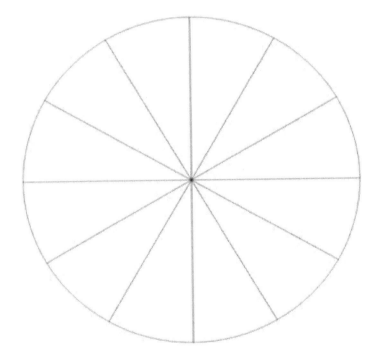

You deserve your best! Go for what you Love!

"Infinite Patience creates immediate results..."

<u>My Walk in Balance Life MAP (FINAL)</u>
(Fill In below...)

<u>Name</u>   Date

I. My Mission – Dream is:

II. Intentions

<u>Intention</u>	<u>Nourish Action</u>	<u>Why</u>
<u>1</u>		
<u>2</u>		
<u>3</u>		

<u>III. My Daily Walk in Balance Wellness Practices, to support me in feeling energized & great</u> (no matter what):

1

2

3

Friday...at Lunch...

Sybrian: Hi, Mac! Did you finish reading the book?

Mac: Yep. I love the Summary. Great stuff in that part!

Sybrian: And...?

Mac: I feel like something's missing.

Sybrian: Like what?

Mac: It's been great having you talk with me and work with me through this, but...

Sybrian: But...?

Mac: I don't know. You've been a great support through it all, but still, something is just 'not there'.

Sybrian: I have a suggestion. I think I know what's missing.

Mac: Well, what is it?

Sybrian: Remember how you said Betty was teasing you about your meditation?

Mac: Yes...

Sybrian: Maybe it's time for you to bring her into your new world so she can Walk in Balance with you! Hasn't she noticed the difference in you? You are happier, more joyful, feeling better physically...don't you want to share that with her?

Mac: I don't think she'd be very interested.

Sybrian: You mean, you're afraid she won't accept the idea. That's your LS talking again. Fear.

Mac: Will that ever stop?

Sybrian: Nope. But you will learn to recognize it when it's happening and then you will do the "STOP –CHALLENGE-CHOOSE" exercise, right then, as it's happening. It's pretty cool when you are able to do that.

Mac: Actually, I did it the other day when I started getting frustrated with a co-worker. I was able to shift my perspective by recognizing my control drama, stopping, and choosing another way of dealing with him. It worked great.

Sybrian: Since it worked so well there for you, don't you think Betty would benefit from learning all of this? Don't you want her to feel as great as you do and to experience more joy?

Mac: I suppose so.

Sybrian: So, share it with her.

Mac: You mean, once I've dealt with my LS fears of rejection and ridicule and shifted into wanting to share with her out of love.

Sybrian: I'm sure she's noticed the changes in you, right?

Mac: Yep. She talks about it quite a bit, actually.

Sybrian: I don't see why she would reject something that has obviously worked for you. Do you?

Mac: You know, you're right! I should share it with her tonight!

Sybrian: I think you'll get even more out of it once you are sharing it with her. It'll be great for both of you! It will make it easier for you to stick to your Core Practices too.

Mac: That's something I didn't think about. Would you mind helping me guide her through?

Sybrian: Not at all! We can start building a brand new "Walk in Balance" tribe and meet in your garden retreat! How is that coming along, by the way?

Mac: We've started the fish pond and waterfall. I expect we'll have the fire pit ready in time for the new moon.

Sybrian: Oh, really?

Mac: Yep. I checked out some of the new moon ceremonies and I actually like the idea of a lot of it. I understand them now.

Sybrian: Awesome!

Mac: How about you come over and join us?

Sybrian: As long as I don't have to see you dancing around the fire in your skivvies, I'd love to!

Mac: I promise, no skivvies dances. Now, after I talk to Betty and we start her on the Core Practices, I guess that's it, right?

Sybrian: Only if you want it to be.

Mac: You mean, there's more?

Sybrian: Oh, yes. Let's get Betty started, if she wants to do this. Then we can move forward after you get a little more practice in and start building our HS, LoA, Walk In Balance Tribe.

Mac: Sounds like a great plan! I can hardly wait!

Chapter 7: Walk in Balance - Summary

Today as I was finishing this book, I had this brainstorm during my session with Coach and I felt connected to this idea of giving myself full permission to enjoy life; an important awareness. Haven't we all suffered too much by trying to live by other people's beliefs and standards? Isn't it time for another way? How about Ethical Hedonism? Awesome! So needed, so good to enjoy life.

It is so important to merge these apparent opposites: the ultimate ethical person of honor and the ultimate person of delight, embracing healthy pleasures, loving, and feeling good. Can they live as one where we are enjoying life to the maximum in a way that is nourishing, wholesome, good, and harms no one yet uplifts all who care to be inspired? Yes!

My whole life I have struggled with my wholesome desires vs. the "should, the must, and have to do" running my mind. I have been at war with myself. Is it this or that, good or bad, and I was always in conflict.

Then I thought, "why not let go of all those tyrannical rules and embrace more fun?" I can trust, right? God has me. My heart and soul is guiding me. So what am I waiting for? Isn't it time for all of us to embrace our heart's truest desire and live! Live the unique expression in our true heart, without asking for anyone's approval. Yes!

Final Exercise: Healing the Blocks to Total Joy Meditation.

Sit quietly, pray and enter presence - and then when ready think deeply about the concept of "absolute fun all day long" for ten minutes. Let yourself focus fully. Breathe it in, make it playful fun and wild how great life can be. Then witness, scan your body for any tightness, pain or stiffness. Meaning: as you focus on joy, any part of you in rebellion will yell. This is **resistance** (which happens whenever you introduce an enlightened new thought-way).

Call forth your heart and with the energy of universal love in you, engulf all the screams, aches, and pains of this resistance. This may manifest as a sore back, the screaming hip, the stiff neck, the headache, and so on. Go there, put your hand on it, and feel it, with your hearts Love full on (light a great light) and let the light of love melt it away.

Observe all that is happening with love and compassion, no fixing or running. Just be. Be with it all during this ten-minute process, and let it simply melt away. Journal anything you become aware of during this process, and when done, you will feel a shift into peace which is your signal to you it is time to relax for a while. Easy eh?

You just gave yourself a gift of your true self, another kind of presence exercise where love conquers all. You see, all those aches are years of accumulated "should do, must do, and have to do" beliefs that have been weighing you down. Let them go. Let love take its place, and with this love give yourself permission to live your life with total delight.

All day long, you live in truth, beauty, and fun...and everyone wins. Nothing is lost and you gain everything. This is the new world from the inside out, from love.

There will be times when you will encounter pain, hurt and "bad things" out in the world. Living a life of joy and love doesn't mean life is always rosy or you ignore issues.

When you encounter something bad out there or you need to take care of or someone you know who is down or hurting, because you are living from your HS, you are better able to deal with these things.

You will be able to help others because you have been mindful of taking care of yourself first. Of course, be authentic, empathize, help, and be there for them. What is the greatest gift you could give the world: Your own happy, loving, joyful heart, right?

The Higher Self in you is total love, compassion, and JOY! The HS is capable of sitting in the fire with anything that happens, and remains to be love. This is the gift of the human experience; the Great Spirit gives us, to practice a wonderful gift of who we really are (love) while being in a place of paradox: beauty and disgust, pleasure and pain, bliss and fear.

Let Us Declare:
I intend to revel in the delight and pleasure of playful loving fun in a way that blesses me and the whole world in joy. Now is the Time, Onward we go...

Letting it go and Letting it come
I have no plan for my life
I accept the plan life has for me
I follow that plan and what it provides me moment to moment
I am not the roles I play in following the plan
I am the witness of all that I interact with in my life
I was a child, an adult, and will soon be an old man.
I was son, a brother, a husband, a father, and a grandfather.
I was an artist, a businessperson, a yogi, a guru, a friend.
I have been healthy, sick, successful, a failure, awake, and asleep.
Behind all those changing experiences, I am the changeless consciousness that is constantly present.
I am that I am, in spite of the changes in that 'I am' experiences.
I am that.
My present is pregnant with all my past.
My future unfolds from the way I live my present
My being manifests in the present
I am present
I am at home in the eternal now, living the plan life has for me.

-Amrit Desai

From Bill:

I have written this book because my heart nudged me to awaken and write down for me and my friends the wisdom I have learned and share it. I write for me. It is not about what others do. It is about what 'I' do from soul, HS.

Love is the answer. And love ignites a fire inside. A fire that says I will not stop until the Love of Great Spirit takes me. I will never quit. I may rest from time to time but never give up. I am here to Be Me, to shine!

Together, we are to become the souls of light we came here to be. This is our highest possible achievement, our most rewarding adventure. Be who you came here to be. Fulfill your destiny. Drop the ego's drama and ask your Great spirit to guide you, protect you, and lead you to your true self. Give up all the fear, and find your way to happiness!

This is a time of great acceleration. We all can know the truth and live it. By living in HS, you motivate others to do the same. Then, love and integrity reign. The peace on earth we have always envisioned will be here.

I know that together many of us are creating a new world by who we are becoming. I pray that my words have inspired you to do so too. Blessings, I salute you!

Mitakuye Oyasin (we are all related in love)

~ Bill

Please send any questions or comments: To:
bill@walkinbalance.org
sybrian@walkinbalance.org

Keys to Remember!

"I know who I AM and what I Want."

"I Create My Life Map and live from there."

ACCEPT AND CREATE

- Meditate each morning, even if just a few minutes. Journal at the end.
- Affirm, Pray, Focus.
- Do Yoga! Or Pilates, Tai Chi, etc., to fill up your tank.
- Take Care of you: Energize Often.
- Exercise regularly.
- Relax your mind.
- Garden.
- Go for a walk in nature.
- Eat good healthy food. Drink LOTS of water.
- Enjoy. Make work play.
- Passionately express your gifts! Play music! Paint! Draw!
- This is your day to love. Make the most of it.
- Touch someone's life, particularly your own.
- Have fun!
- Teach: Unity (connection), Energy (vitality), and Impeccability (focus, honor) to all!

Promise Yourself

"Promise yourself
To be so strong that nothing can disturb your peace of mind.

To talk health, happiness, and prosperity to every person you meet.

To make all your friends feel that there is something special in them.

To look at the sunny side of everything and make your Optimism come true.

To thInk only of the best, to work only for the best, to be the best, and expect only the best.

To be just as enthusiastic about the success of others as you are about your own.

To forget the mistakes of the past and press on to the greater achievements of the future.

To wear a cheerful countenance at all times and give every living creature a smile.

To give so much to the improvement of yourself that you have no time to criticize others.

To be too large for worry, too noble for anger, too strong for fear, and too happy to permit the presence of trouble."

- Christian. D. Larson

Journey to the Mountain top

Dear Creator:

Help me to open my eyes to beauty, to wonder, to meaning, to appreciate your miracles.
Help me to understand and know my relationships to other creatures;
To accept myself and others as you have made them.
Help me to seek hope, imagination, joy, wisdom, inner peace.
May I go forth under the open sky and listen to nature's teachings.
Slow me down, Lord! There is more to life than increasing speed.
Life is not a race, but a dance, and the music can end any time.
Because I am going to die, I must not forget how to live!
Time can be fast or slow, full or empty, meaningful or wasted.
I should deliberate and take time to follow my dreams.
Let me value each day and know eternity.
Let me see your spirit in every place.
By looking both inward and outward, I can realize my sense of worth.
Help me too look into the night skies and search the stars for understanding.
Let me look into my heart and spirit for love and goodwill.
Help me to associate with creative and caring people, wherever I may find them.
And know those people of peace and freedom who can change the world.
Through wilderness, we remember and are brought home again.
Life is eternal. We are a part of something infinite and fundamental.
May I be the most complete person I can possibly be, to live, to feel, think, and dream. And may I never forget where I can from and how precious a gift, life is.

- R. Baron and T. Locker

As I Walk with Beauty

As I walk, as I walk
The universe is walking with me
In beauty it walks before me
In beauty it walks behind me
In beauty it walks below me
In beauty it walks above me
Beauty is on every side
As I walk, I walk with Beauty.

- *A Traditional Navajo Prayer*

"Now faith is the substance of things hoped for,
the evidence of things not seen."

- *Hebrews 11:1 King James Version (KJV)*

*"The Great Spirit doesn't put a dream in your heart without
giving you the power to make it come true.
The catch is, you might have to work for it."*

- *Major L. Roy Lynch - Campfire Talks*

The Invitation

It doesn't interest me what you do for a living. I want to know what you ache for, and if you dare to dream of meeting your heart's longing. It doesn't interest me how old you are. I want to know if you will risk looking like a fool for love, for your dream, for the adventure of being alive.

It doesn't interest me what planets are squaring your moon. I want to know if you have touched the center of your own sorrow, if you have been opened by life's betrayals or have become shriveled and closed from fear of

further pain! I want to know if you can sit with pain, mine or your own, without moving to hide it or fade it, or fix it.

I want to know if you can be with joy, mine or your own, if you can dance with wildness and let the ecstasy fill you to the tips of your fingers and toes without cautioning us to be careful, to be realistic, to remember the limitations of being human.

It doesn't interest me if the story you are telling me is true. I want to know if you can disappoint another to be true to yourself; if you can bear the accusation of betrayal and not betray your own soul; if you can be faithless and therefore trustworthy.

I want to know if you can see beauty even when it's not pretty, every day, and if you can source your own life from its presence.

I want to know if you can live with failure, yours and mine, and still stand on the edge of the lake and shout to the silver of the full moon, "Yes!"

It doesn't interest me to know where you live or how much money you have. I want to know if you can get up, after the night of grief and despair, weary and bruised to the bone, and do what needs to be done to feed the children.

It doesn't interest me who you know or how you came to be here I want to know if you will stand in the center of the fire with me and not shrink back.

It doesn't interest me where or what or with whom you have studied. I want to know what sustains you, from the inside, when all else falls away.

I want to know if you can be alone with yourself and if you truly like the company you keep in the empty moments.

- Oriah Mountain Dreamer

My thanks to my mentors for the use of their quotes

Invocation/Benediction: *Bill O'Mara*

Wild Geese, Mary Oliver (and the Journey)
http://www.rjgeib.com/thoughts/geese/geese.html

I will not live and unlived Life, Dawn Markova, online 2013.

Decide to go for it: Boldness has Genius, *William Hutchinson Murray* (1931-1996) from his book titled "The Scottish Himalayan Expedition", page 8.

Quotes: 2007 by *Bill O'Mara* Three quotes

The Path *Tim Walking Bear*, by permission

The Peace of the Wild Things: *Wendell Berry* from *The Selected Poems of Wendell Berry.* Copyright © 1998

Promise Yourself: *Christian D. Larson, Page 118.*
http://cornerstone.www.hubs.com/larson.html

"Letting it go and Letting it Come". *Amrit Desai,* as quoted from the book by Stephen Cope, Yoga and the Quest for the True Self, *page 303. 2000 Bantam, New York*

Journey to the Mountain Top: by *R. Baron and T. Locker,* poem from the book, "Journey to the Mountain Top"

The Invitation, *Oriah Mountain Dreamer, copyright (1999) Page,121.*

Campfire Talks, *Maj. L. Roy Lynch, by permission*

<u>References</u>

Andrews, Ted (1993). *Animals Speak*. Llewellyn. St. Paul, Minnesota.

Bear, Sun & Wabun. (1992). *The Medicine Wheel: Earth Astrology*. Fireside Books. New York.

Bear, Sun, Mulligan, C. Nurfer, P, and Wabun (1989). *Walk in Balance*. Prentice Hall. New York.

Chopra, Deepak (1994). *The 7 Spiritual Laws of Success*. New World Library. San Rafael, California.

Csikszentmihalyi, M. (1990). *Flow*. Harper Perennial. New York.

Covey, Stephen (1989). *The 7 Habits of Highly Effective People*. Fireside. New York.

Dyer, Wayne W. (2002). *10 Secrets for Success and Inner Peace*. Hay House. Carlsbad, California. (2003). *The Power of Intention*. Hay House. Carlsbad, California.

Forest, Ohky Simine (2000). *Dreaming the Council Ways*. Weiser. York Beach, Maine

For Your Improvement: A Development and Coaching Guide. Lominger. 612.542.1466

Frankl, V. (1984). *Man's Search for Meaning*. Pocket Books. New York:

Gawain, Shakti (1995). *Creative Visualization*. New World Library. Novato, California.

Gerber, Michael (1998). *The E-Myth Manager.* Harper Collins. New York.

Gray, John (1980). *What You Can Feel, You Can Heal.* Heart books. San Francisco.

Harner, M. (1990). *The Way of the Shaman.* Harper and Rowe. San Francisco.

Hay, Louise (1987). *You Can Heal your Life.* Hay House. Carlsbad, California.

Hawkins, David R. (2002). *Power Vs. Force.* Hay House. Carlsbad, California.

Katie, Byron. (2002). *Loving What Is: Four Questions That Can Change Your Life.* Harmony Books. New York

King, S. K. (1990). *Urban Shaman.* Fireside. New York.
Luthans, F. (1995). *Organizational Behavior.* McGraw Hill. New York.

Maffetone, Phil. (1989). *In Fitness and In Health.* Barmore Productions. Stamford, New York.

Millman, D. (1993). *The Life you were Born to Live.* HJ Kramer. Tiburon, California.

O'Mara, Bill (2000). *The Godspell Solution.* Granite Publishing. North Carolina.

O'Mara, Bill (2003). *The Way of the Corporate Shaman.* San Diego, CA: Corporate Shaman Press.

Peale, N. V. (1952). *The Power of Positive Thinking.* Fawcett Publications. Greenwich, Connecticut., (1987). *A Different Drum.* Simon and Schuster. New York.

Peters T. J. and Waterman, R.H. *In Search of Excellence: Lessons from America's best-run companies.* Harper & Row. New York

Quirk, P. E. (1993). *When Spirits meet the Red Path.* Northwest. Salt Lake City, Utah. (1994)., *The Vision.* Woodlands Press. Salt Lake City, Utah.

Redfield, James (1993). *The Celestine Prophecy.* Satori Press. Hoover, Alabama.

Robbins, Anthony. (1986). *Unlimited Power.* Ballantine Books, New York.

Roman, Sanaya (1986). *Living With Joy.* H.J.Kramer. California.---. (1986). *Power Through Awareness.* H.J.Kramer. California.---. (1989). *Spiritual Growth.* H.J.Kramer. California.

Ruiz, D. M. (1997) *The Four Agreements.* Amber Allen. San Rafael, California.

Senge, P.M., (1990). *The 5th Discipline. The Art and Practice of the Learning Organization.* Doubleday/Currency. New York.

Slater, Robert (1999). *The GE Way Fieldbook: Jack Welch's Battle Plan for Corporate Revolution.* McGraw-Hill. New York.

Successful Managers Handbook. Personnel Decisions International 1-800.633.4410.

Storm, Hyemeyohsts (1972). *Seven Arrows*. Ballantine. New York.

Tolle, Eckert (1999). *The Power of Now*. New World Library. Novato, California.

Vigil, Bernadette (2001). *Mastery of Awareness*. Bear and Company. Rochester, Vermont.

Wilde, Stuart (1987). *Affirmations*. Hay House. Carlsbad, California.

Wilde, Stuart (1998). *The Little Money Bible*. Hay House. Carlsbad, California.

Williamson, Marianne (1993). *A Return to Love*. Harper Perennial. New York.

Whitehouse, William (2009). The Magician's Way: What It Really Takes to Find Your Treasure. New World Library, Novato, California.

Suggested Reading List

In addition to <u>Walk in Balance,</u> we recommend the following books for further learning.

Progressive Business books

The Way of the Corporate Shaman by O'Mara
The Path of the Enlightened Leaders by O'Mara
The 7 Habits of Highly Effective People by Stephen Covey
Principle-Centered Leadership by Stephen Covey
Flow (and Flow at Work) by M. Cisentmikahly
The E-Myth Manager by Michael Gerber
The Fifth Discipline by Peter Senge
Primal Leadership by D. Goleman, Boyatzis, & McKee
The Art of Happiness at Work by H.H. The Dalai Lama
The One-Minute Manager by Blanchard & Johnson
In Search of Excellence by Peters
Mastery by George Leonard
Management of the Absurd by Richard Fardson
The Power of Purpose: Creating Meaning in Your Life and Work by Richard Leider
1001 Ways to Reward Employees by Nelson
The 10-Day MBA by S. Silbiger
Tao of Leadership by John Heider
Zen at Work by Les Kaye
Corporate Mystic by G. Hendricks
Stewardship by Peter Block
Up Against the Wal-marts by Taylor and Archer
West Point Leadership Lessons by Scott Snair
The Greatest Salesman in the World by Og Mandino

Classics in Spiritual reading:

The Godspell Solution by B. O'Mara
OverComing, When Tough Times Happen by B. O'Mara
The Power of Positive Thinking by Norman Vincent Peale
The Celestine Prophecy by James Redfield
A Course in Miracles – Foundation for Peace

Spiritual Growth by Sanaya Roman
Living in Joy by Sanaya Roman
Personal Power through Awareness by Sanaya Roman
The Seven Spiritual Laws of Success by D. Chopra
All books by J. Krishnamurti.
All books by Stuart Wilde
All books by Marianne Williamson
The Way of the Peaceful Warrior by Dan Millman
The Power of Now by Eckhart Tolle
Creative Visualization by S. Gawain
You Can Heal your Life by Louise Hay
The Power of Intention by Wayne Dyer
Illusions: The Adventures of a Reluctant Messiah by Richard Bach
Mastery of Awareness by Dona Bernadette Vigil
Walk in Balance, The Medicine Wheel, and others by Sun Bear
The Wind is My Mother, The Life & Teachings of a Native American Shaman by Bear Heart
The Way of the Shaman by M. Harner
Urban Shaman by S. K. King
Animals Speak by Ted Andrews
The Four Agreements by D. M. Ruiz
Dreaming the Council Ways by Ohky Simine Forest
Black Elk Speaks by Black Elk
Medicine Woman by Lynn Andrews

Other Resources

Holistic Healing Centers:

Kripalu Center   www.kripalu.org

The Center for Shamanic Studies   www.shamanism.org

The Dance of the Deer Foundation   www.shamanism.com

The Ojai Foundation   www.ojiafoundation.org

The Findhorn Foundation   www.findhorn.org

Harbin   www.harbin.org

Vision Quest School   http://www.schoolofnaturalwonder.org

Leadership Centers:

Corporate Shaman Way   www.corporateshamanway.com

CFLG   www.thecentreforleadershipgroup.com

The Center for Creative Leadership   www.leaders.ccl.org

The Man-Kind Project   www.mkp.org

Ken Blanchard Co.   www.blanchardtraining.com

Personnel Decisions International
www.personneldecisions.com

Franklin-Covey   www.franklincovey.com

Peter Senge   www.infed.org/thinkers/senge.htm

Music for the Soul:

www.PeaceThroughMusic.com

www.rootlight.com

www.spiritatwork.com:

Spirit at work is an association dedicated to those professionals involved with spirituality in the workplace. The association offers retreats, workshops, conferences, local chapter meetings and a newsletter. In addition, you will find chat rooms and discussion forums available. Spirit in business practitioners are listed as well.

Appendix

The summary of 'The Way' from "The Way of the Corporate Shaman" book. Available on Amazon.com

A Shaman's Plan for Life:
The Shaman's Vision: Discovering your true self and living this self fully: learning, healing, loving, and serving.

The Shaman's Purpose: Living the Sacred Way. This means living the Seven Principles, Accepting & Creating, Letting Go, Allowing and Embracing, living in harmony with the Law of Attraction, following your inner guidance, and using the healing techniques outlined here to serve yourself so that you may better serve the Whole.

A.) Inner Peace:
1. Set aside daily sacred **time; be alone to center in spirit, in quiet, in nature, where you can practice prayer, listening and accepting all as perfect.** Meditate, sitting in total silence, quieting the mind, and embracing your Higher Self. There are many ways to meditate, counting breaths, watching a candle, listening to a recorded guided meditation tape, repeating a phrase or mantra. Find a class or teacher from whom you can learn some of these invaluable practices.

2. Celebrate the sacred: **Participate in sacred ceremonies,** alone and in groups. Find a drumming circle; take part in a Prayer Pipe ritual. Create sacred spaces in your home, using precious objects, pictures, stones, plants, or shells. Buy a musical instrument and play it. Buy a sage bundle and light it, and bless your space with its sacred smoke. This ancient native practice of "smudging" is amazingly effective for cleaning the energy and blessing people, places, and things.

3. Love someone each day, even if that means something as simple as smiling at them from your heart, telling the truth with compassion for their feelings, or offering to walk their dog. Share love, share of yourself.

4. Watch for signs, for there is **guidance** all around you. It may come on the wind... in a hawk flying overhead... in the serendipitous coincidences of your life. Pay attention to your dreams and bursts of intuition.

   Arrange to go on **a Vision Quest**: Take an extended Journey for guidance with the support of a trusted shaman.

B.) Purification and Energizing: Purify Your Body

1. Engage in **daily movement** or exercise: walk, bike, or practice yoga, tai chi, or martial arts.

2. Sweat to **release toxins**. Take part in a sacred native Sweat Lodge. If that is not available to you take hot salt or mineral baths, or a sauna. BREATHE deeply.

3. Maximize **Nutrition:** Eat mostly green, organic live foods, and appropriate proteins. Drink lots of water. Find a nutritional consultant to advise you regarding herbs that will be helpful for you. A good read here is Dr. Phil Maffetone's, "In Fitness and In Health."

4. **Listen to your body's needs.** Eat in a sacred way. Bless your food, (i.e.) "Thank you for surrendering your life, my friend, so that I may continue mine." Take your time. Chew each bite (30) times. Much of

our stomach and digestive problems occur from 'scarfing' down food and not eating in a sacred way. Fast for a week (under supervision).

C.) Purifying Your Mind and Emotions:

1. Be still in your mind. **Take time to meditate** throughout the day, and take part in support groups to help you drop the need to control and to assist you in clearing and releasing the past. Smudge with sage daily to clear your energy field. Be quiet inside. Develop awareness.

2. **Reframe** your unconscious habits and reactions. Find a new perspective to replace the thoughts that hurt. Affirm what you want, by transforming blame and reaction into acceptance and self-empowerment. Don't assume that you know what others mean by what they say, and never take anything personally. Move from sloppy, disorganized living to being impeccable in your actions and with your word. (See The Four Agreements by Don Miguel Ruiz for more on this).

3. **Always be Accepting and Creating.** Accept what is, and from the place of acceptance let your Higher Self guide you to create what you need. Use the Ultimate Transformation Formula (Chapter 3) when you are emotionally triggered. Let go of pain. Forgive and release each day. Create life the way you see it.

D.) Purifying Your Spirit:

1. Go on a **Shamanic Journey** (as outlined earlier in Chapter 5) to find your "power animal" and receive

guidance. Your power animal will bring you a message or a healing and make clear your next steps.

2. Receive **Energy Work**. We are made of energy. Go to a Reiki healer, or a healer who uses other Light or Sound Energy healing methods. Focus on and nurture your own life energy.

3. **Take part in sacred circle groups and celebrations**. Dance, sing, celebrate, share, listen, and enjoy drumming & music with others. Gentle healing sound is wonderfully healing. Chant 'Om' and 'Ah' slow, repeatedly and feel what happens to your body.

4. Experience a **Soul Retrieval,** a process In which a healer guides you into an altered state of awareness to find your power animal, release past trauma, and take back your power.

5. As needed, a **Shamanic Healing or Extraction**, a guided process with a healer to release negative energies and disease from the body.

Disclaimer:
This book, should not be considered, in any way,
to replace sound professional medical or
psychological consultation and/or treatment.

About the Author(s)

William O'Mara, Ph.D., has been a pioneer in the personal growth movement and has been for many years one of America's most gifted spirit leadership teachers.

He is president of the Centre for Leadership Group. O'Mara is an external director of leadership training for a major hotel company. He has an advanced degree in Psychology as well as certifications in Neuro-Linguistic Programming and Holistic Health, and he is a Reiki Master.

His book, *The Godspell Solution*, is a modern day philosophical classic. His last book, *The Way of the Corporate Shaman*, is a breakthrough in the genre of spirituality in business.

He has led workshops, retreats, and gatherings all over the USA for the past 15 years sharing his business expertise and the native American wisdom he learned during his time with the renowned native American "spirit caller" Speaking Wind.

He is an award-winning corporate speaker and is available by request for select speaking engagements, coaching and consultations.

Contact Information*: bill@walkinbalance.org*

Other Works by Bill:

The Path of the Enlightened Leader(s)
The Way of the Corporate Shaman
The Godspell Solution - a Journey
Walk In Balance - Life Energy E-Book
Overcoming - When Tough Times Happen – Finding Happiness

Sybrian Castleman has worked for many years as a Leadership, Customer Service, Sales, and Team Building Coach. She is a Life Coach and is a Trainer in various soft skills. Much of her work has been through leadership positions with volunteer organizations such as: Kiwanis International, Girl Scouts, and the USAF Auxiliary/Civil Air Patrol where she is currently serving as a Squadron Commander.

Through these organizations and many others, she has worked with adults and youth to develop leadership skills, build positive self-images, and help them discover their own internal resources in overcoming challenges.

Sybrian is a Reiki Master, Certified Public Speaker, Corporate Trainer, and holds many additional certifications in various areas. She has led workshops and provided individual coaching to many individuals. Her "10 Day Baby Steps" workshop has been touted as highly successful for participants. Sybrian is available for coaching and workshops.

Contact Information: *Sybrian@walkinbalance.org*

Other works by Sybrian:

The Ten Day Baby Step Challenge
The Magic of Being Extraordinary (middle school level)

Thank you for reading Walk in Balance.

->***Ask Us about Shift Coaching, to apply the lessons of this book In Your Life.*** www.walkinbalance.org 760-809-4478

Made in the USA
Lexington, KY
27 January 2016